SUPER EASY PREDIABETES

DIET AND ACTION PLAN

40-Day Meal Guide with Low-GI Recipes, Nutrition Tips, and Lifestyle Strategies to Balance Blood Sugar and Support Lasting Health

DR KURT WASHINGTON

Copyright Page

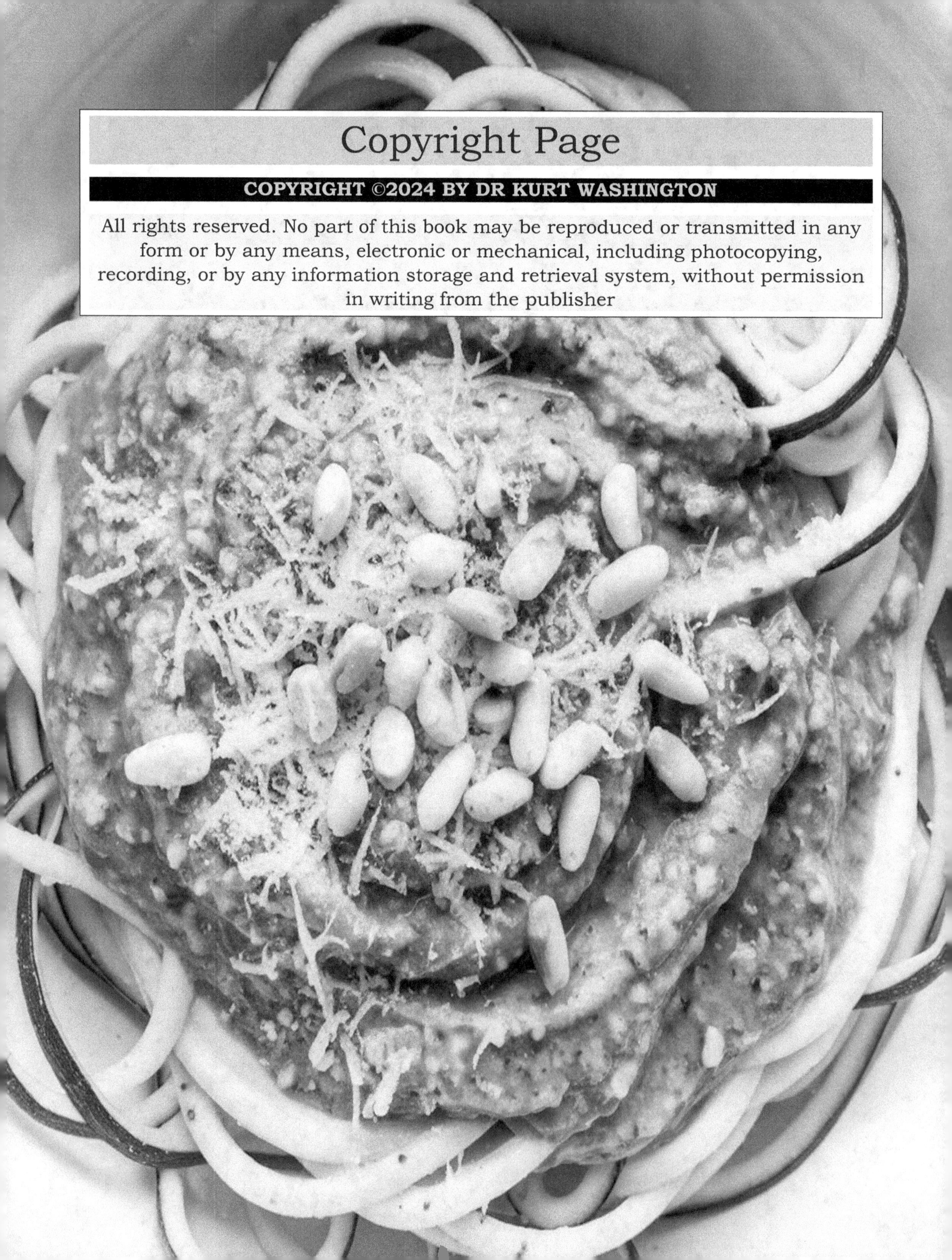

TABLE OF CONTENT

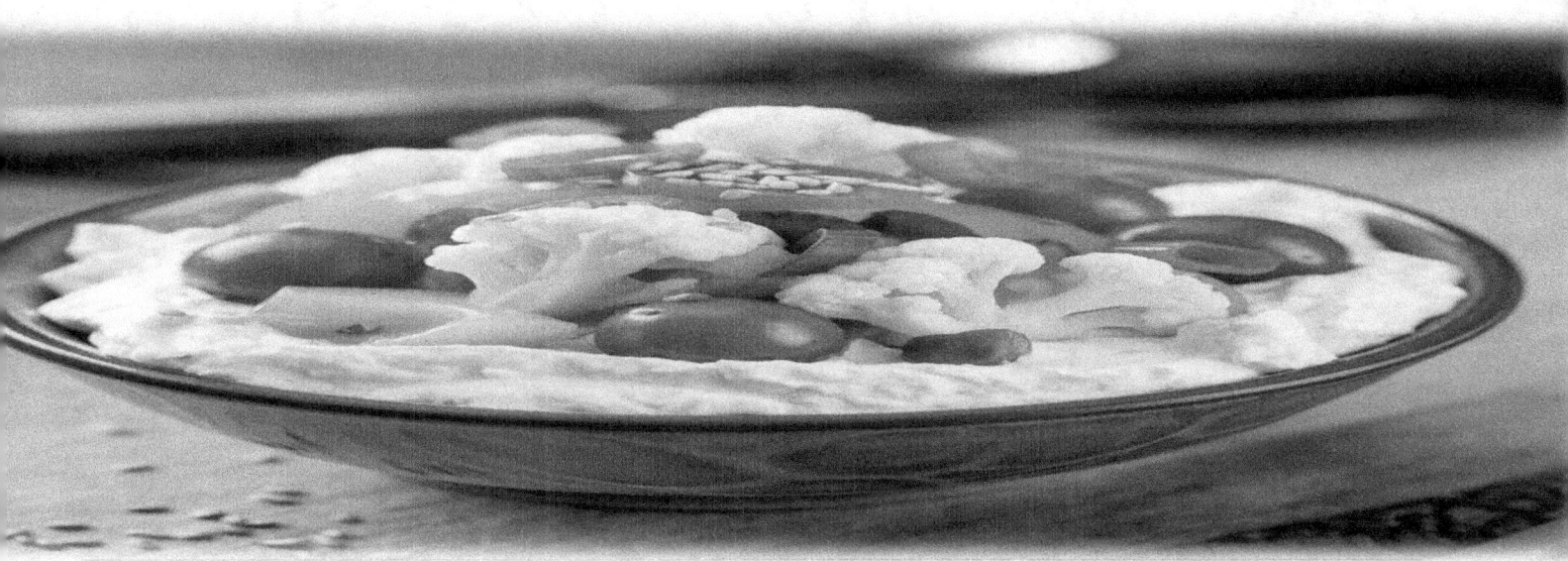

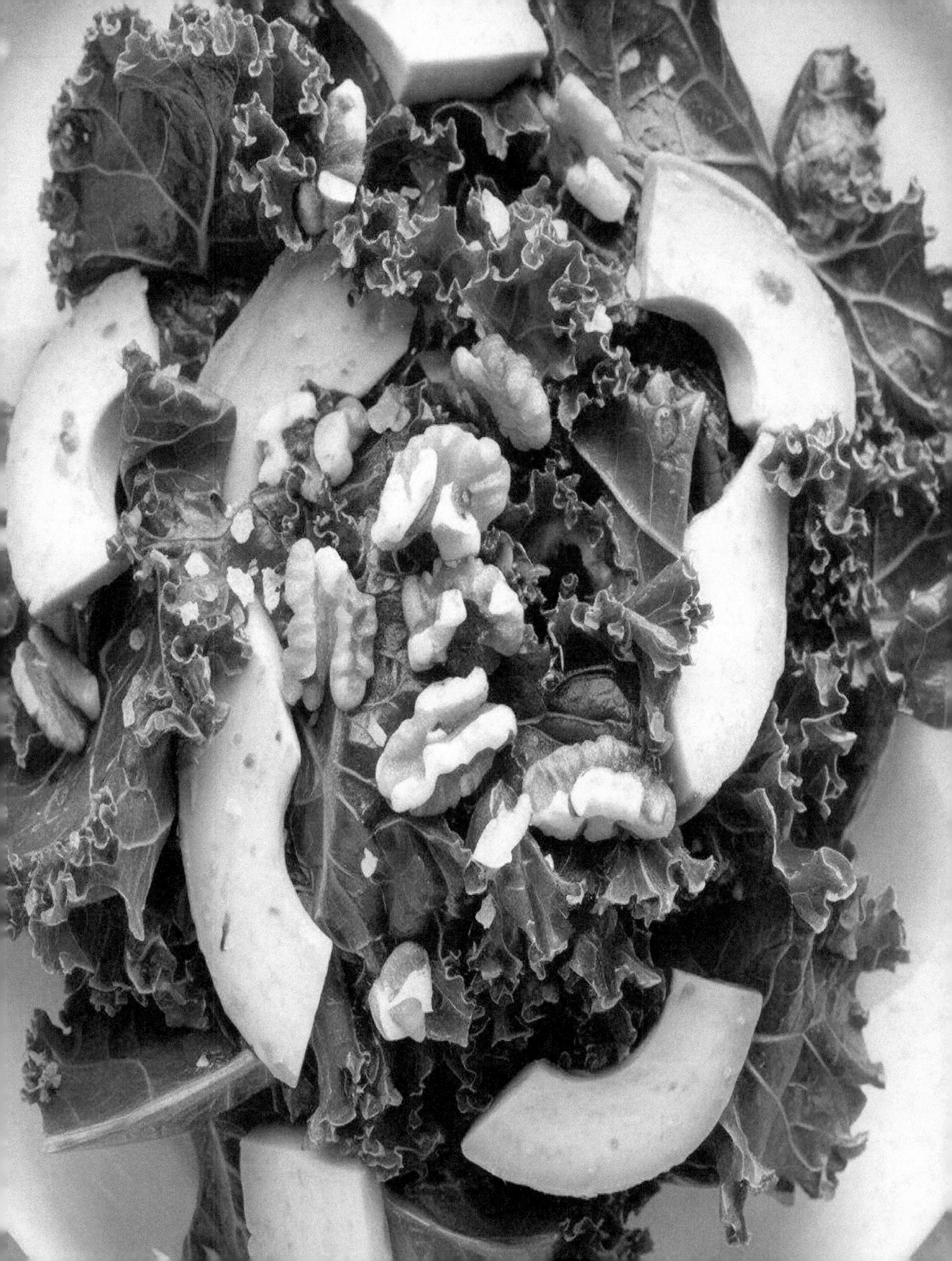

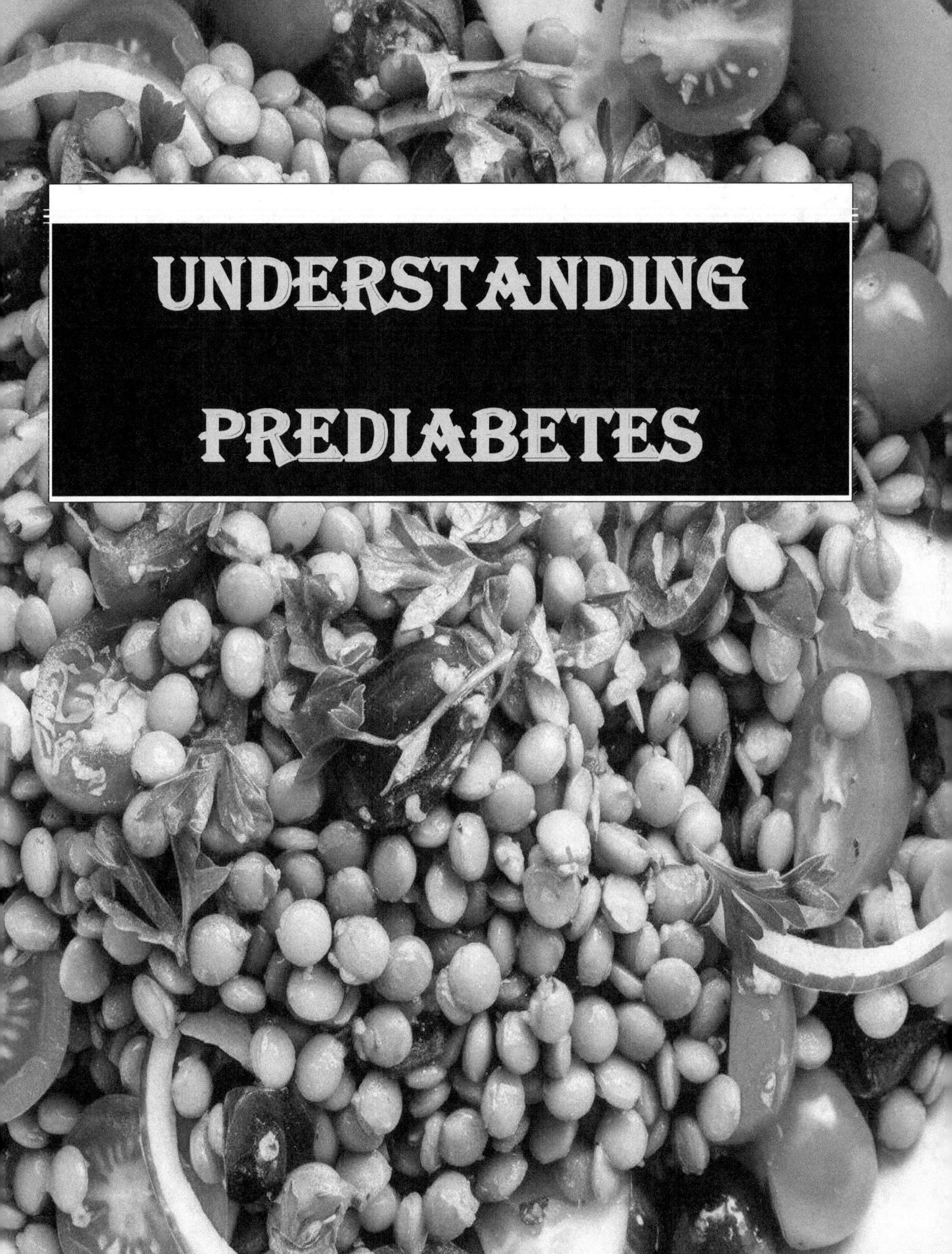

UNDERSTANDING

PREDIABETES

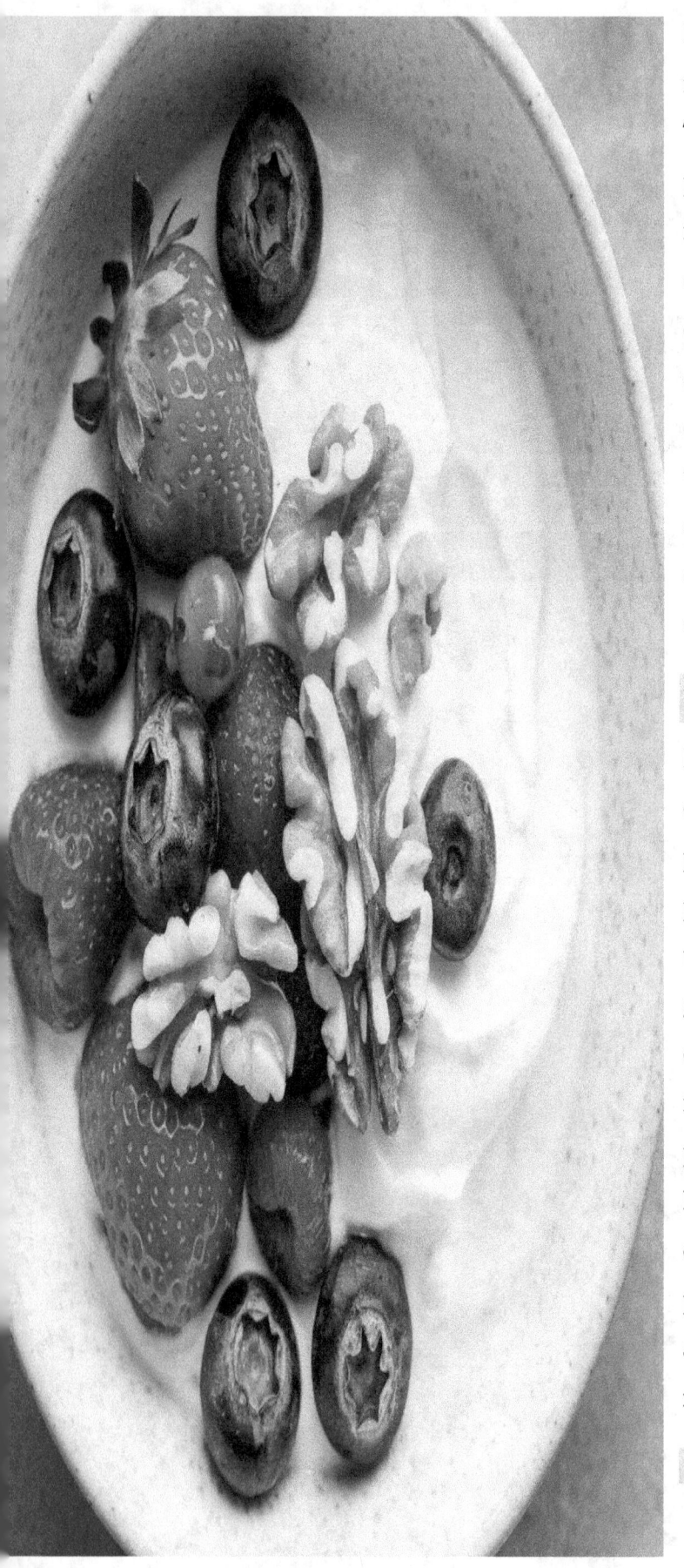

Elevated blood sugar levels that are above normal but not high enough to qualify as Type 2 diabetes are the hallmark of prediabetes, a metabolic disorder. It is an important indicator that your body is starting to experience insulin resistance, a disorder in which cells in your body lose their sensitivity to the hormone insulin, which controls blood sugar levels. It is impossible to overestimate the significance of identifying and treating prediabetes since it offers a chance to take action before diabetes and its consequences develop.

In contrast to diabetes, which is characterized by insufficient insulin production or inefficient use of the insulin produced, prediabetes is characterized by the body's continued ability to regulate glucose levels, but at a level that is cause for concern. Untreated prediabetes can develop into Type 2 diabetes, a dangerous illness that poses a number of health hazards, such as kidney damage, nerve damage, heart disease, and visual issues. By being aware of prediabetes, you can adopt a better lifestyle and take preventative measures to avoid more issues.

- Knowing your individual risk profile is crucial since a number of factors might raise your chance of having prediabetes. The following are a few typical risk variables that are relatable and easily accessible:

- Family History: The risk of prediabetes can be significantly influenced by genetics. You are more likely to acquire prediabetes if you have a parent or sibling with diabetes. Being aware of your family's medical history might assist you maintain your health awareness.

- Weight: One of the biggest risk factors is being overweight, especially if the extra weight is distributed around the belly. Insulin resistance may be exacerbated by the hormones produced by fat cells, particularly those found in the abdominal region.

- Physical Inactivity: Your risk of developing prediabetes is greatly increased by a sedentary lifestyle. Frequent exercise lowers blood sugar, increases insulin sensitivity, and aids in weight control. Movement, even in tiny doses, can have an impact.

- Age: As people age, particularly after the age of 45, their risk of developing prediabetes rises. Our bodies may become less adept at using insulin as we age because our metabolisms naturally slow down.

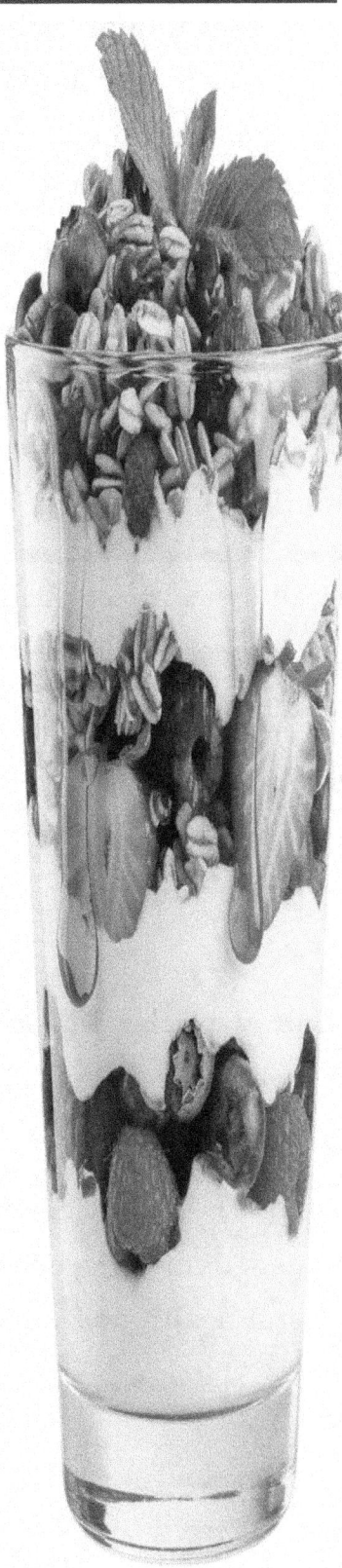

- Ethnicity: Some ethnic groups are more likely to develop Type 2 diabetes and prediabetes than others, such as Native Americans, African Americans, Hispanic Americans, and some Asian Americans.

- Gestational Diabetes: You are more likely to acquire prediabetes in the future if you had gestational diabetes throughout your pregnancy. This can be a crucial moment for women to keep a closer eye on their health after giving birth.

- High Blood Pressure and Low HDL Cholesterol: You are more likely to develop insulin resistance and prediabetes if you have high blood pressure (more than 130/80 mmHg) or low HDL cholesterol.

You can more accurately evaluate your circumstances and reduce your risk by being aware of these risk variables.

Implications for Health

Serious health consequences may result from neglecting to treat prediabetes. The development of Type 2 diabetes, which impacts millions of people and can result in life-altering complications, is the most worrisome danger.

Progression to Diabetes: Research indicates that if treatment is not received, people with prediabetes have a 15% to 30% chance of becoming Type 2 diabetes after five years. The importance of changing one's lifestyle at a young age is highlighted by this statistic.

Cardiovascular Risks: A higher risk of heart disease and stroke is frequently linked to prediabetes. High blood sugar can raise triglyceride and cholesterol levels, which increases the risk of artery-clogging plaque.

Kidney Damage: Chronic kidney disease or kidney failure may result from high blood sugar's damaging effects on the kidneys' blood vessels. Serious consequences for general health and wellbeing may result from this.

Nerve Damage: Neuropathy, which results from uncontrolled blood sugar levels, can cause pain, tingling, and numbness in the hands and feet. As the illness worsens over time, mobility problems and a decreased quality of life may result.

Vision Issues: Serious eye disorders such diabetic retinopathy, which can cause vision loss, are more likely to develop in those with prediabetes. These problems can be avoided with early detection and treatment.

Cognitive Decline: Recent studies indicate a connection between prediabetes and cognitive decline, which includes a higher chance of developing dementia, including Alzheimer's disease.

Motivating lifestyle changes requires an understanding of the possible health hazards linked to untreated prediabetes. You can take control of your health and make decisions that can result in a healthier, diabetes-free future by being aware of your risk factors and the consequences of prediabetes.

In summary, prediabetes is an urgent call to action rather than only a diagnosis. The good news is that prediabetes can be reversed and the risk of Type 2 diabetes can be considerably decreased with early intervention, lifestyle modifications, and regular monitoring. Armed with information and resolve, embrace this path to a healthy way of living.

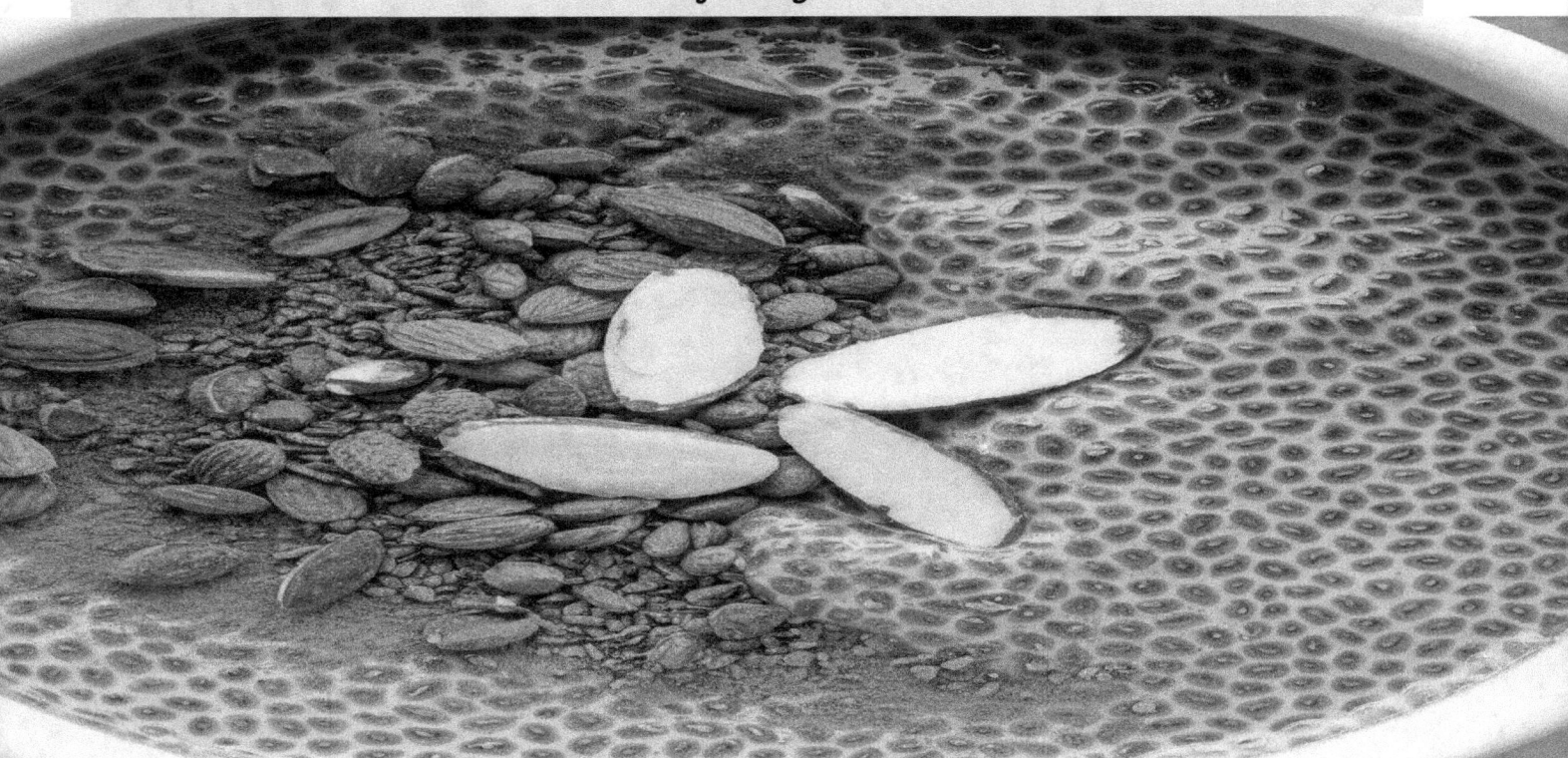

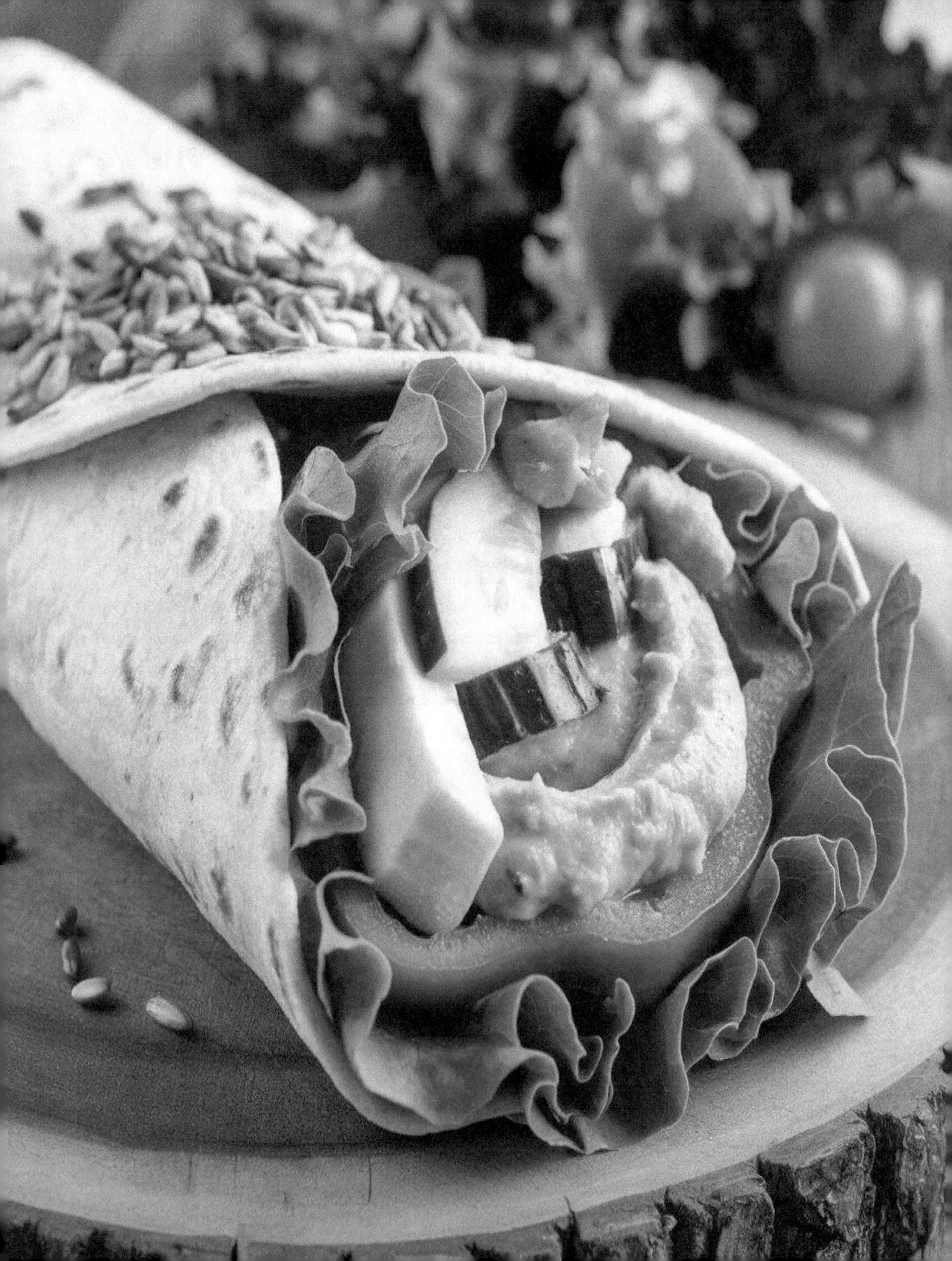

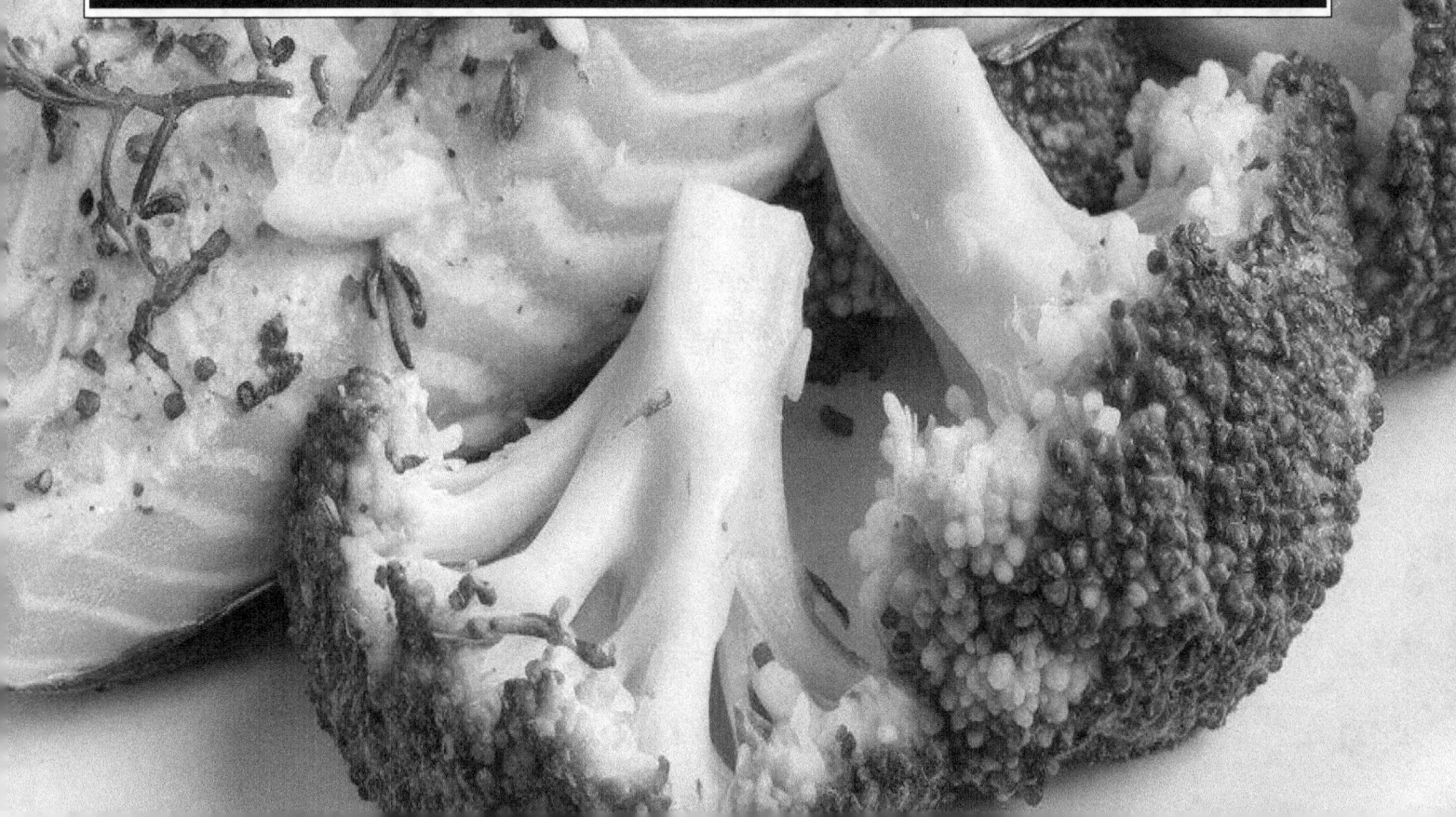

NUTRITION'S FUNCTION IN THE MANAGEMENT OF PREDIABETES

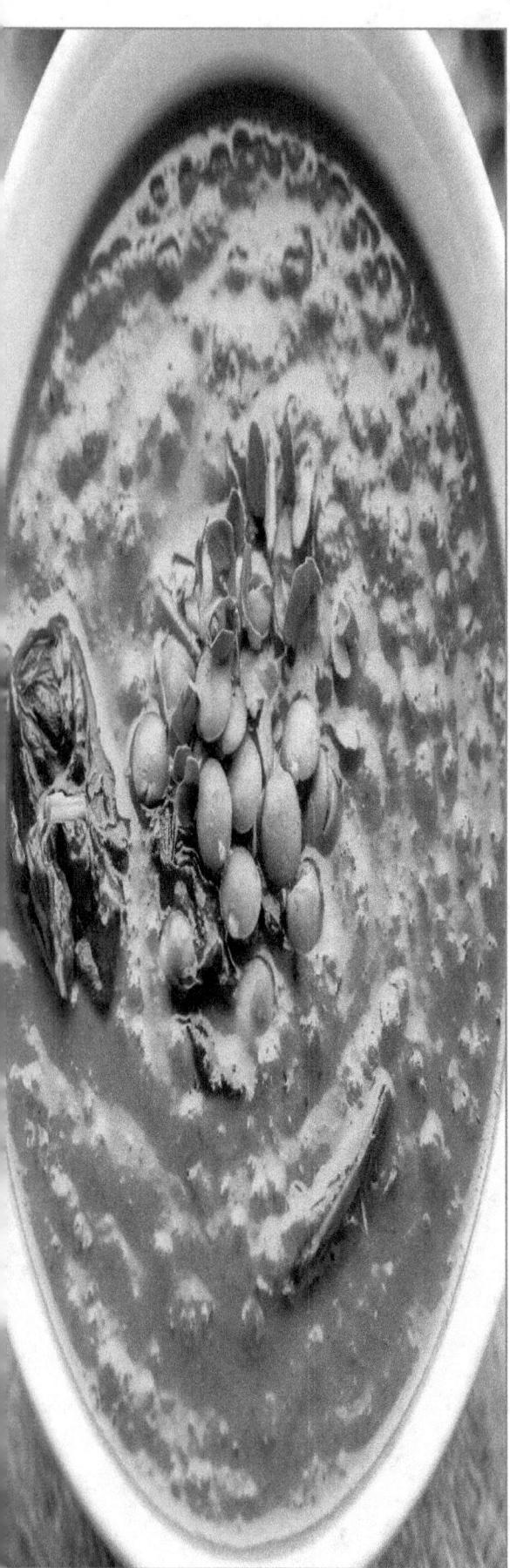

The Value of a Well-Balanced Diet

A key component of managing prediabetes is nutrition. In addition to providing vital nutrients, the foods we eat directly affect blood sugar levels. Making educated food choices becomes crucial when managing prediabetes. A balanced diet lowers the chance of developing Type 2 diabetes, encourages weight loss, and helps maintain stable blood sugar levels.

Carbohydrates, proteins, fats, vitamins, and minerals are all part of a balanced diet. Each is essential for sustaining vitality, promoting physiological processes, and guaranteeing general health. By knowing how to blend these food types, one can make meals that efficiently control blood sugar levels while nourishing the body.

Carbohydrates: Making Sensible Choices

When talking about diet and blood sugar, carbohydrates are frequently the main topic of conversation. The fact that not all carbohydrates are made equal must be understood. Complex carbs, such as those found in whole grains, legumes, fruits, and vegetables, are digested more slowly and give longer-lasting energy than processed carbohydrates, which can induce sharp rises in blood sugar.

Brown rice, quinoa, and whole wheat bread are examples of whole grains that can help balance blood sugar levels. Because of their high fiber content, these grains slow down digestion and the bloodstream's absorption of glucose.

Fruits and veggies: Make sure your diet includes a range of vibrant fruits and veggies. They offer vital minerals, vitamins, and antioxidants that promote general well-being. Their fiber content can also help control blood sugar levels and facilitate digestion.

Legumes: Chickpeas, lentils, and beans are great providers of fiber and protein. They are an excellent option for blood sugar stabilization because of their low glycemic index.

Portion Control: It's critical to comprehend portion quantities. Excessive consumption of even healthy carbohydrates might raise blood sugar levels. To control portions, use visual cues (such as your fist or palm as a guide) or measurement devices.

Proteins: Essential Components of Health

Maintaining muscle mass, encouraging fullness, and regulating blood sugar levels all depend on protein. You can manage prediabetes and promote general health by include a range of protein sources in your diet.

Lean Proteins: Select lean meats with less saturated fat, like fish, poultry, and turkey. Omega-3 fatty acids, which are abundant in fish, especially fatty types like salmon, have been connected to heart health.

Plant-Based Proteins: Include sources of plant-based protein include nuts, seeds, tempeh, and tofu. These include fiber and good fats in addition to protein.

Dairy and Substitutes: A healthy diet can include low-fat dairy products like milk and yogurt. To stay away from added sugar, choose low-sugar or unsweetened options.

Good Fats: Not All Fats Are Created Equal

Although they should be chosen carefully and consumed in moderation, fats are an essential component of a balanced diet. Good fats can increase satiety, lower inflammation, and strengthen the heart.

Include foods high in unsaturated fats, such as nuts, seeds, avocados, and olive oil. These fats offer necessary fatty acids that are good for general health and can lower cholesterol.

Limit Saturated and Trans Fats: Steer clear of trans fats, which are present in a lot of processed and fried meals, and cut back on saturated fats, which are present in red meat, butter, and full-fat dairy. These fats have the potential to elevate heart disease risk and cholesterol levels.

Preparing Meals for Prediabetes

Meal planning can make grocery shopping more efficient and guarantee that you always have wholesome selections on hand. The following advice will help you design a diet that is specifically suited to controlling prediabetes:

Every meal should aim for a balanced plate, with half of it made up of non-starchy vegetables, 25% consisting of lean protein, and 25% consisting of whole grains or nutritious carbohydrates.

Make Snacks: Eating wholesome snacks in between meals might help maintain stable blood sugar levels. Think about choices like Greek yogurt with berries, a piece of fruit with a handful of nuts, or raw veggies with hummus.

Keep Yourself Hydrated: Your preferred beverage should be water. Maintaining proper hydration can aid in weight management and is crucial for general health. Fruit juices and sugary drinks should be avoided as they can cause blood sugar increases.

Attempt New Recipes: Don't be scared to attempt new recipes that use the foods that are suggested for prediabetes management. This can make eating healthily sustainable and pleasurable.

Comprehending Food Labels

One of the most useful skills for diet management is learning to read food labels. Making healthy decisions can be facilitated by knowing what to look for:

Serving Sizes: Be mindful of serving sizes to make sure you're not eating more than you planned to.

Total Carbohydrates: Pay particular attention to the amount of sugars and dietary fiber in your diet. Choose foods that are low in added sugars and high in fiber.

Ingredients List: The list of ingredients should be as brief as possible. Select goods with whole, identifiable constituents rather than ones with lengthy lists of fake additives.

The management of prediabetes is mostly dependent on nutrition, and long-term success depends on knowing how to choose healthy foods. You can successfully control your blood sugar levels and lower your chance of developing Type 2 diabetes by emphasizing a balanced diet full of whole foods, keeping an eye on your carbohydrate intake, and paying attention to portion sizes.

Making educated decisions is the first step on the path to improved health. Keep in mind that minor adjustments might result in major gains as you continue to study and use the dietary techniques described in this chapter. Give yourself the information and self-assurance you need, and use nutrition as a tool to help you reach your best possible health.

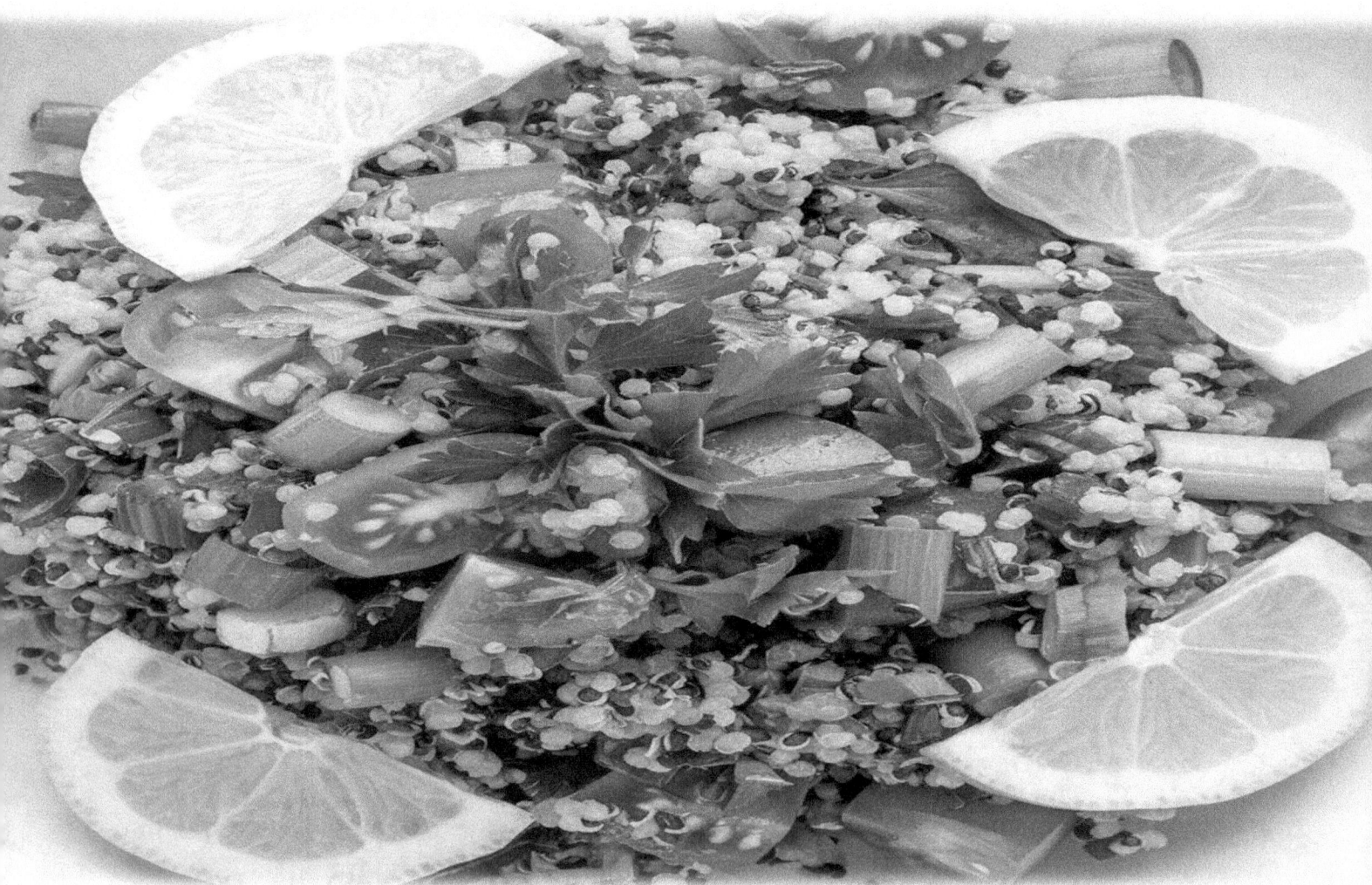

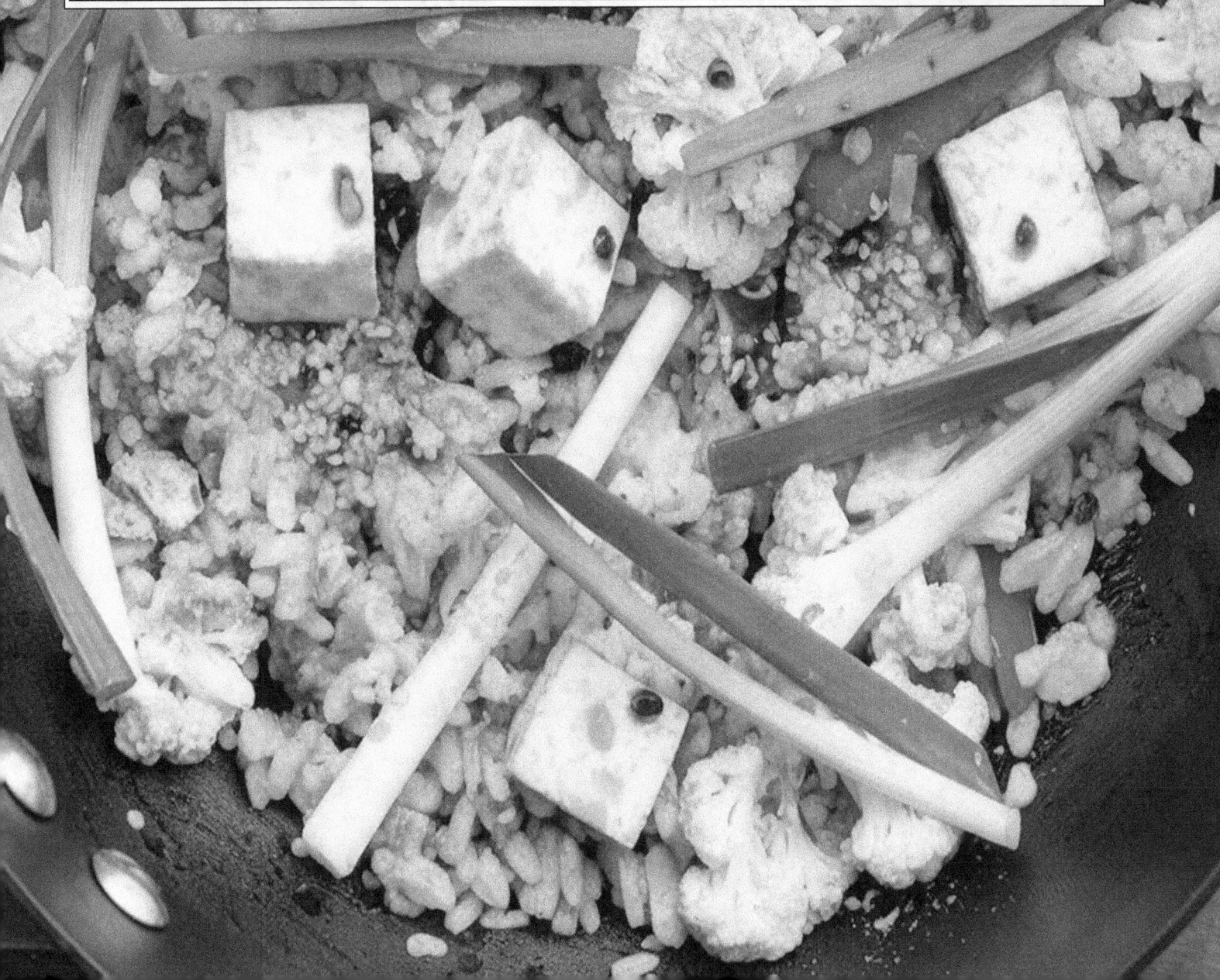

LOW GLYCEMIC INDEX

(GI) DIET

Greek Yogurt and Berry Parfait

Ingredients

- 1 cup unsweetened Greek yogurt

- 1/2 cup mixed berries (blueberries, strawberries, raspberries)

- 1 tablespoon chia seeds

- 1/4 teaspoon cinnamon

Preparation Method

- In a serving bowl, layer half of the Greek yogurt.

- Add half of the berries and sprinkle with chia seeds and cinnamon.

- Add the remaining yogurt and top with the remaining berries.

- Let sit for a few minutes to allow the chia seeds to soften.

Nutritional Value

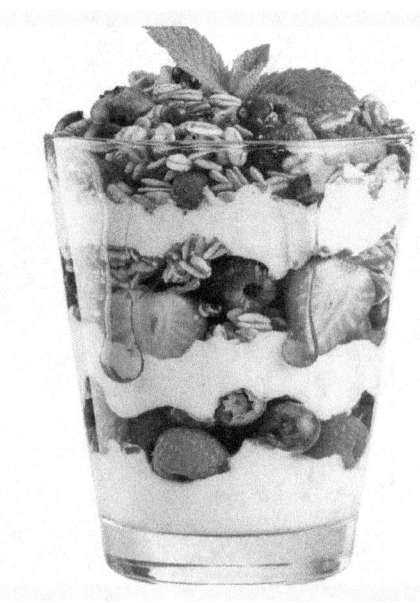

- Calories: 180 kcal

- Protein: 14g

- Carbohydrates: 18g (fiber-rich)

- Fats: 4g

- GI: Low, with balanced carbs and protein

Avocado and Hummus Veggie Wrap

🔘 Ingredients

- 1 whole-grain wrap or lettuce leaves for low-carb version
- 2 tablespoons hummus
- 1/4 avocado, sliced
- 1/4 cup shredded carrots
- 1/4 cucumber, sliced
- 1/4 bell pepper, sliced
- Handful of spinach leaves

🔘 Preparation Method

- Spread hummus evenly on the wrap or lettuce leaves.
- Arrange avocado slices, carrots, cucumber, bell pepper, and spinach on top.
- Roll up tightly, slice in half, and serve.

🔘 Nutritional Value

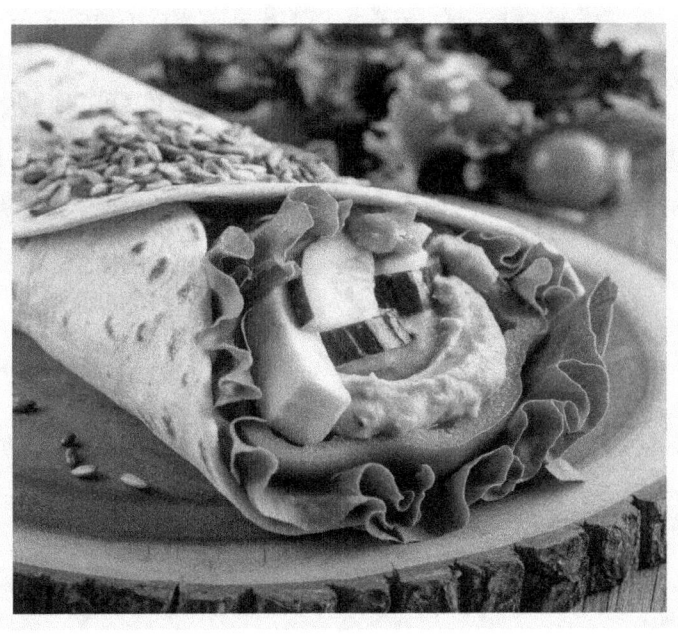

- Calories: 220 kcal
- Protein: 6g
- Carbohydrates: 25g (fiber-rich)
- Fats: 10g
- GI: Low, due to fiber and healthy fats

Lentil and Spinach Soup

⚙ Ingredients

- 1/2 cup dry lentils, rinsed
- 1 tablespoon olive oil
- 1 small onion, chopped
- 1 garlic clove, minced
- 2 cups vegetable broth
- 1 cup spinach leaves
- Salt and pepper, to taste

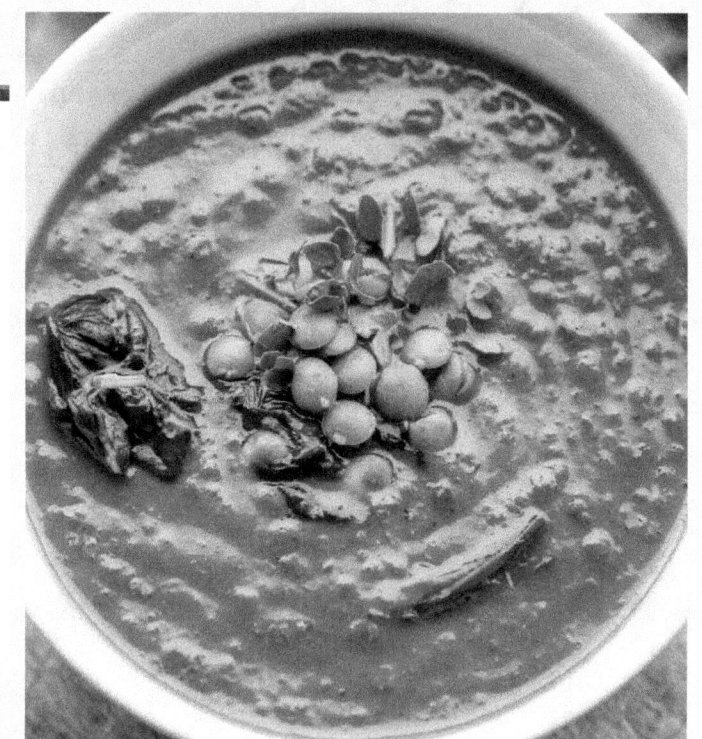

⚙ Preparation Method

- Heat olive oil in a pot, add onion and garlic, and sauté until soft.
- Add lentils and broth; bring to a boil.
- Reduce heat, cover, and simmer for 20-25 minutes until lentils are tender.
- Stir in spinach, season with salt and pepper, and cook until spinach wilts.

⚙ Nutritional Value

- Calories: 180 kcal
- Protein: 10g
- Carbohydrates: 22g (fiber-rich)
- Fats: 4g
- GI: Low, packed with fiber and protein

Quinoa Salad with Chickpeas and Veggies

Ingredients

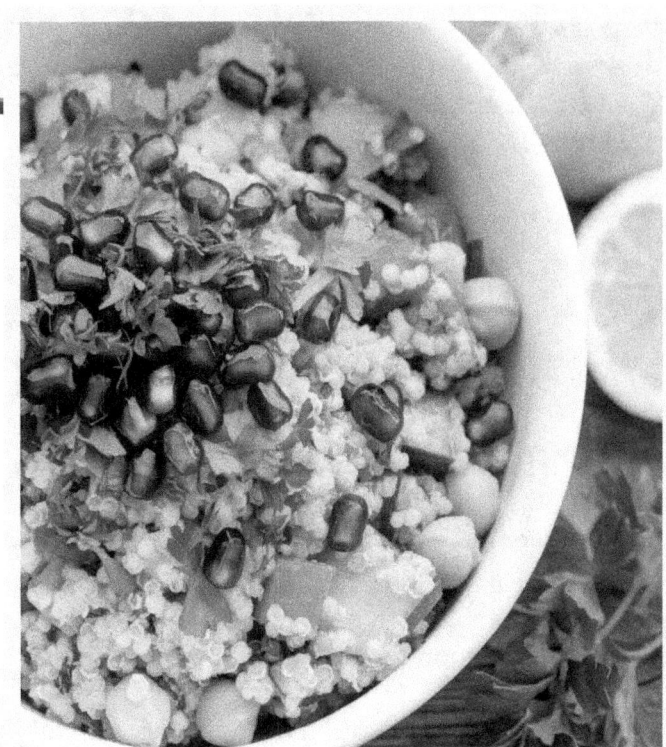

- 1/2 cup cooked quinoa

- 1/4 cup canned chickpeas, rinsed and drained

- 1/4 cup diced cucumber

- 1/4 cup cherry tomatoes, halved

- 1 tablespoon olive oil

- Juice of 1/2 lemon

- Salt and pepper, to taste

Preparation Method

- In a large bowl, combine quinoa, chickpeas, cucumber, and tomatoes.

- Drizzle with olive oil and lemon juice; season with salt and pepper.

- Toss to combine and serve chilled.

Nutritional Value

- Calories: 210 kcal

- Protein: 8g

- Carbohydrates: 30g (fiber-rich)

- Fats: 7g

- GI: Low, with slow-digesting carbs and fiber

Baked Salmon with Steamed Broccoli

Ingredients

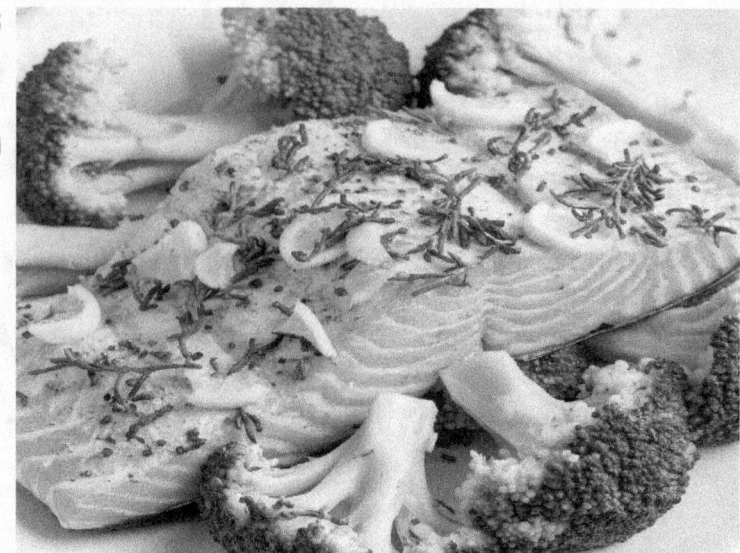

- 4 oz salmon fillet
- 1 cup broccoli florets
- 1/2 tablespoon olive oil
- Salt, pepper, and lemon juice, to taste

Preparation Method

- Preheat oven to 375°F (190°C). Season salmon with salt, pepper, and lemon juice.
- Bake salmon for 15-20 minutes until flaky.
- Steam broccoli until tender and drizzle with olive oil before serving alongside salmon.

Nutritional Value

- Calories: 250 kcal
- Protein: 22g
- Carbohydrates: 6g (fiber-rich)
- Fats: 15g
- GI: Low, due to lean protein and minimal carbs

Cottage Cheese and Vegetable Bowl

Ingredients

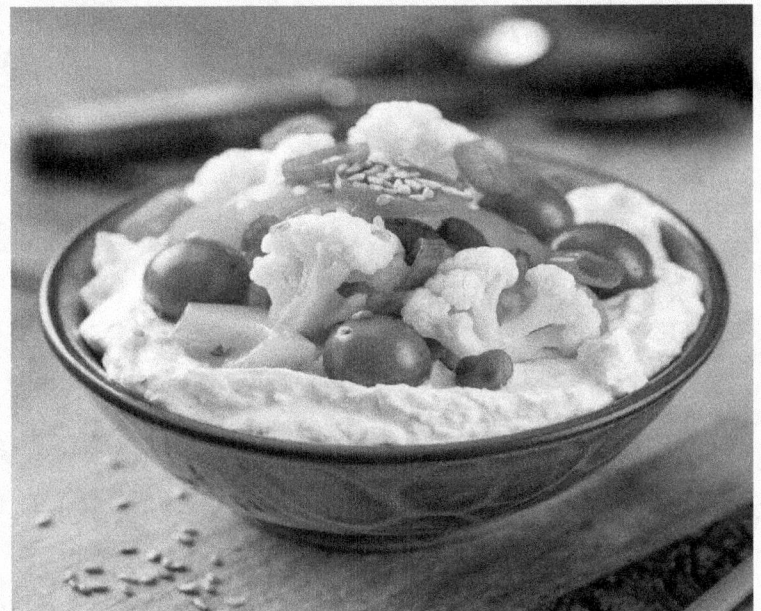

- 1/2 cup low-fat cottage cheese

- 1/4 cup sliced cucumber

- 1/4 cup cherry tomatoes, halved

- 1/4 avocado, sliced

- Fresh herbs (basil or parsley), optional

Preparation Method

- Place cottage cheese in a bowl and arrange cucumber, tomatoes, and avocado around it.

- Sprinkle with fresh herbs if desired and serve immediately.

Nutritional Value

- Calories: 180 kcal

- Protein: 14g

- Carbohydrates: 10g (fiber-rich)

- Fats: 8g

- GI: Low, with lean protein and healthy fats

Spinach and Mushroom Omelet

Ingredients

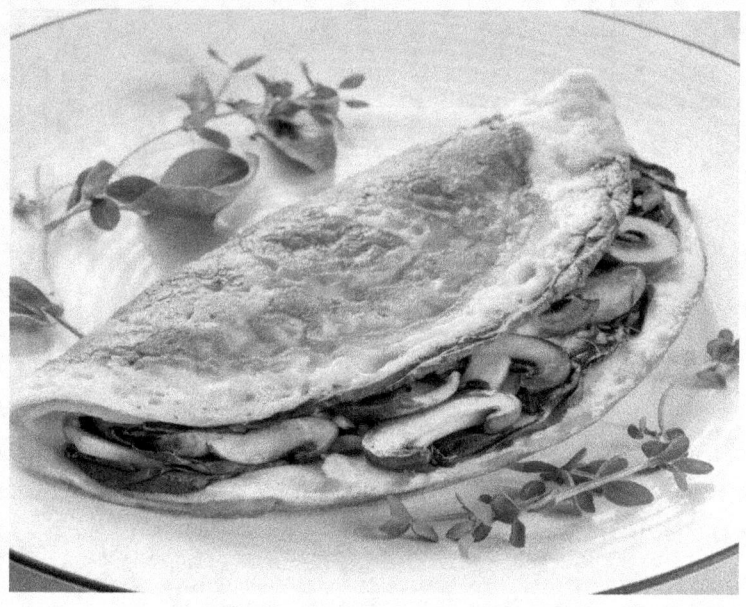

- 2 eggs or 1 egg + 2 egg whites

- 1/2 cup spinach leaves

- 1/4 cup sliced mushrooms

- Salt and pepper, to taste

Preparation Method

- Whisk eggs, add salt and pepper.

- In a non-stick skillet, cook mushrooms until soft; add spinach until wilted.

- Pour eggs over veggies, cook until set, then fold.

Nutritional Value

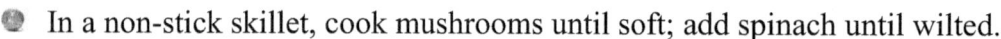

- Calories: 160 kcal

- Protein: 12g

- Carbohydrates: 3g (fiber-rich)

- Fats: 10g

- GI: Low, with high protein

Zucchini Noodles with Pesto

Ingredients

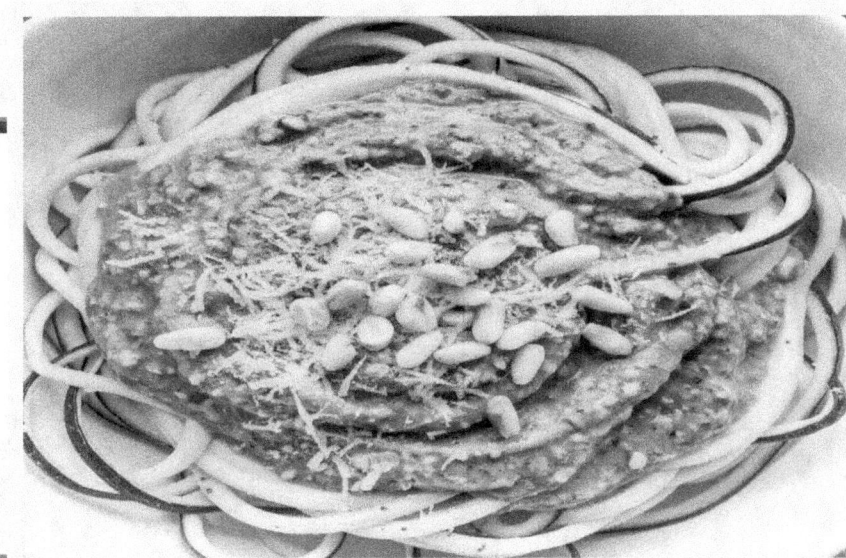

- 1 zucchini, spiralized

- 2 tablespoons pesto sauce

- Cherry tomatoes, for garnish

Preparation Method

- Steam zucchini noodles for 2-3 minutes until tender.

- Toss with pesto sauce and garnish with cherry tomatoes.

Nutritional Value

- Calories: 150 kcal

- Protein: 4g

- Carbohydrates: 10g (fiber-rich)

- Fats: 8g

- GI: Low, with healthy fats

27

Chia Pudding with Almond Milk

Ingredients

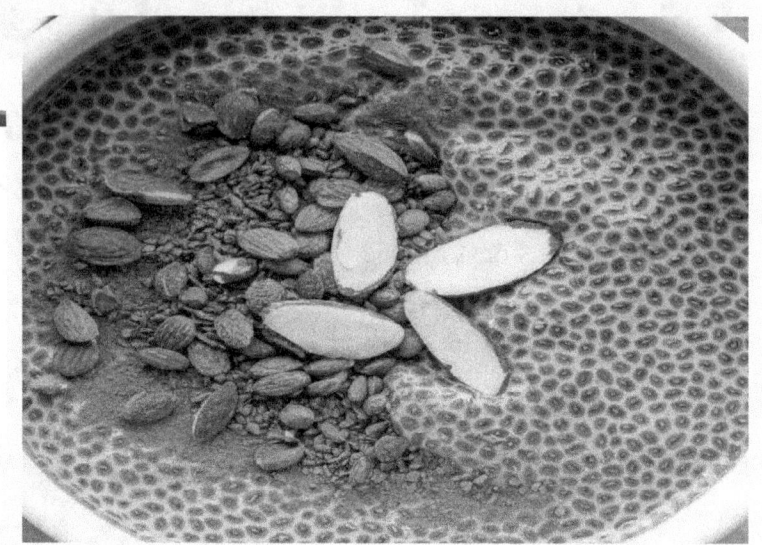

- 1/2 cup unsweetened almond milk

- 2 tablespoons chia seeds

- 1/4 teaspoon vanilla extract

Preparation Method

- Combine almond milk, chia seeds, and vanilla in a bowl.

- Stir well and refrigerate overnight.

- Stir again in the morning and enjoy.

Nutritional Value

- Calories: 140 kcal

- Protein: 4g

- Carbohydrates: 8g (fiber-rich)

- Fats: 9g

- GI: Low, with fiber from chia seeds

Cauliflower Rice Stir-Fry

Ingredients

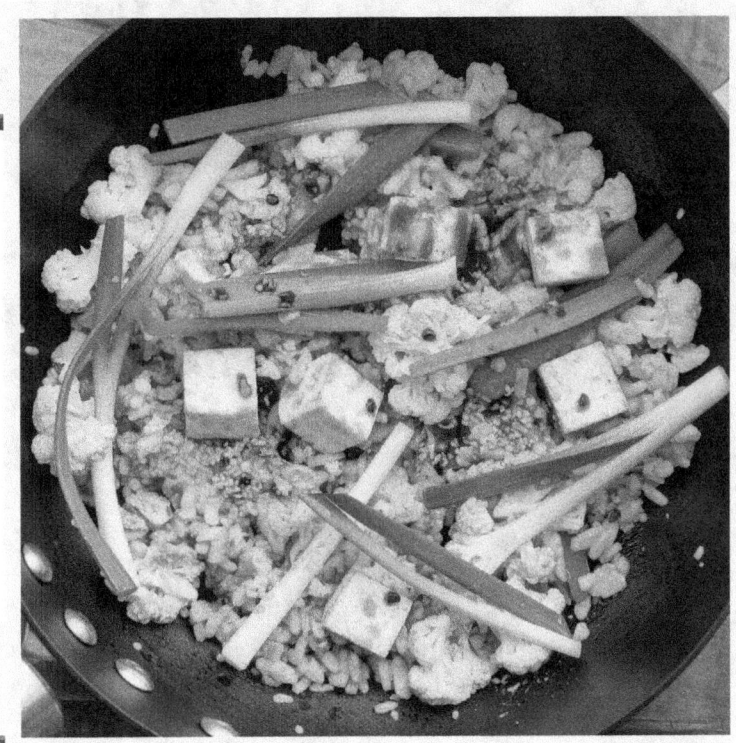

- 1 cup cauliflower rice

- 1/4 cup diced bell pepper

- 1/4 cup peas

- 1 tablespoon olive oil

- Salt, pepper, and garlic powder, to taste

Preparation Method

- Heat olive oil in a pan; add cauliflower rice and bell pepper.

- Sauté for 5-7 minutes, add peas, and season with salt, pepper, and garlic powder.

Nutritional Value

- Calories: 120 kcal

- Protein: 4g

- Carbohydrates: 10g (fiber-rich)

- Fats: 5g

GI: Low, with nutrient-dense veggies

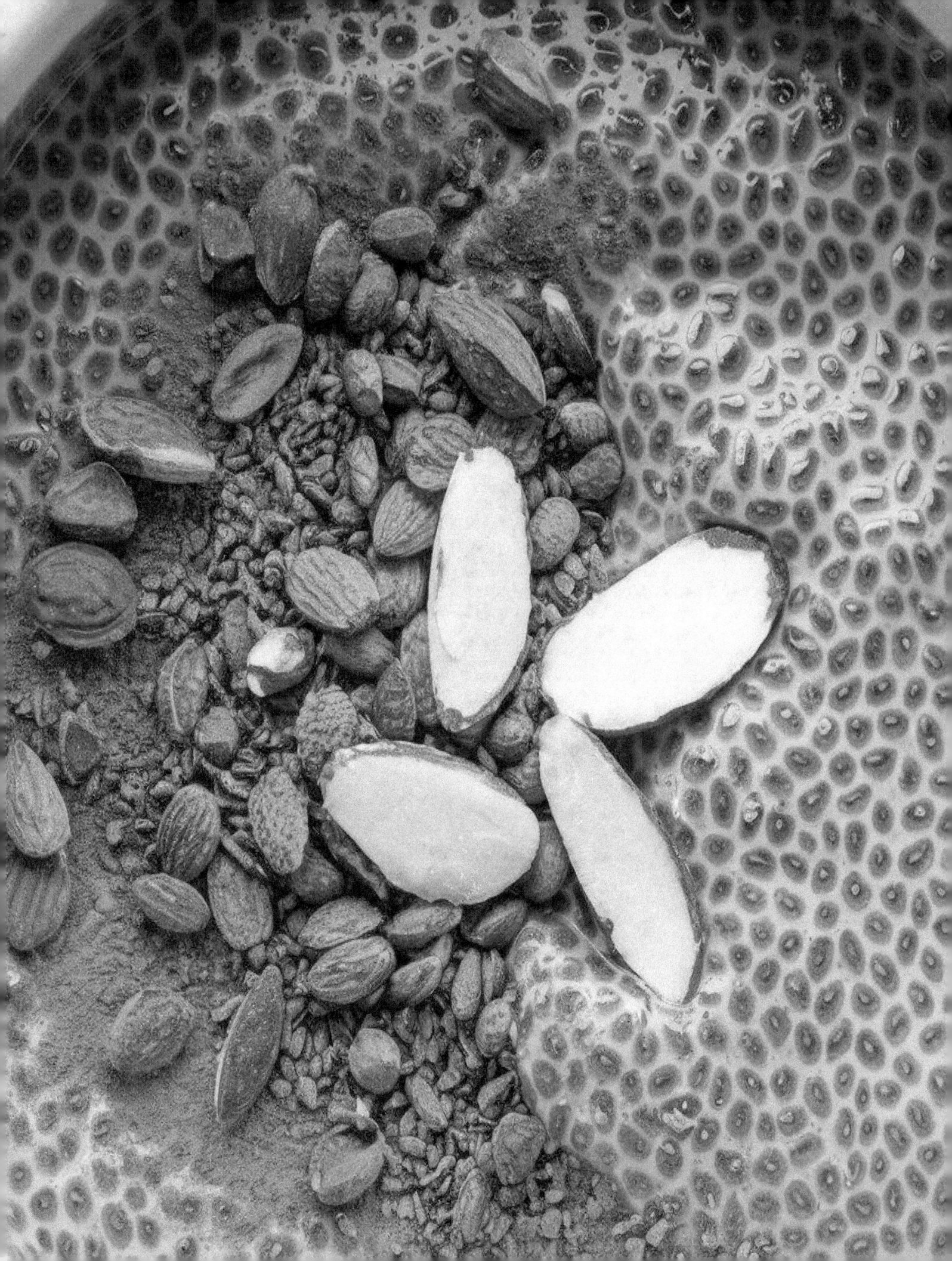

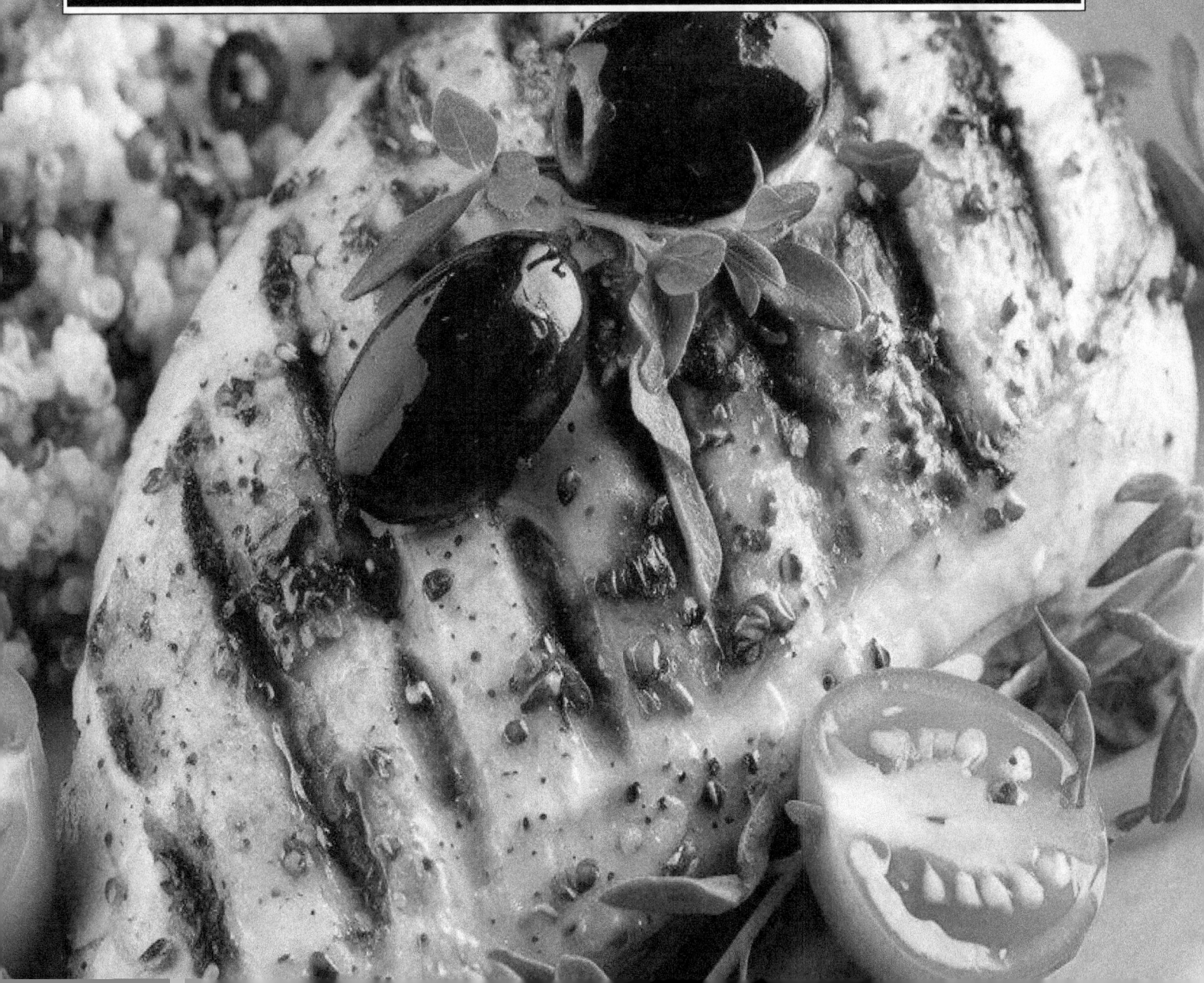

MEDITERRANEAN

DIET RECIPES

Chickpea and Vegetable Salad

Ingredients

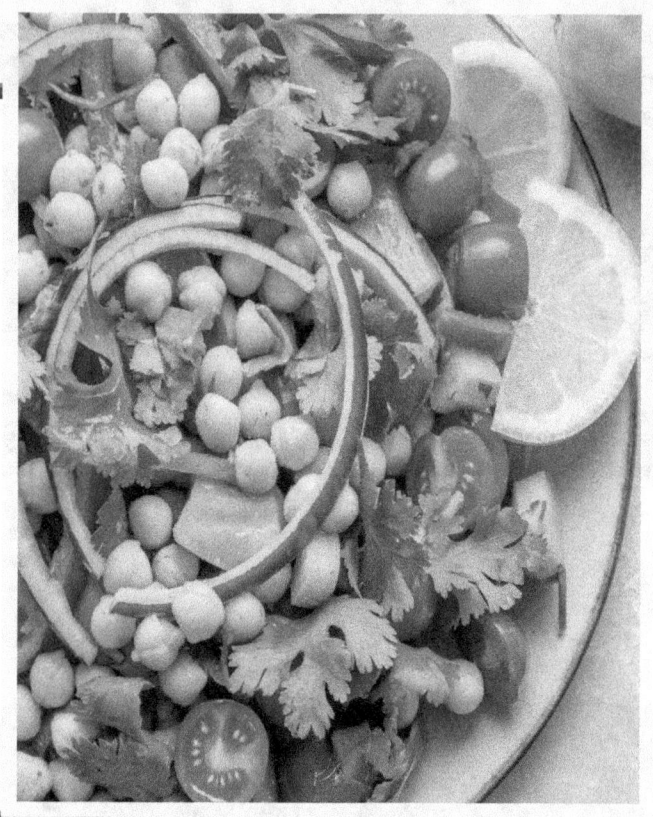

- 1 cup canned chickpeas, rinsed and drained

  1/2 cucumber, diced

  1/2 red bell pepper, diced

  1/4 cup cherry tomatoes, halved

  1/4 cup red onion, finely chopped

  1 tablespoon olive oil

  Juice of half a lemon

  Salt and pepper, to taste

Preparation Method

- In a mixing bowl, combine chickpeas, cucumber, bell pepper, tomatoes, and red onion. Drizzle with olive oil and lemon juice, then season with salt and pepper. Toss well to combine and serve chilled.

Nutritional Value

- Calories: 220 kcal

  Protein: 8g

  Carbohydrates: 30g (fiber-rich)

  Fats: 8g

  GI: Low, with balanced fiber and healthy fats

Mediterranean Grilled Chicken

Ingredients

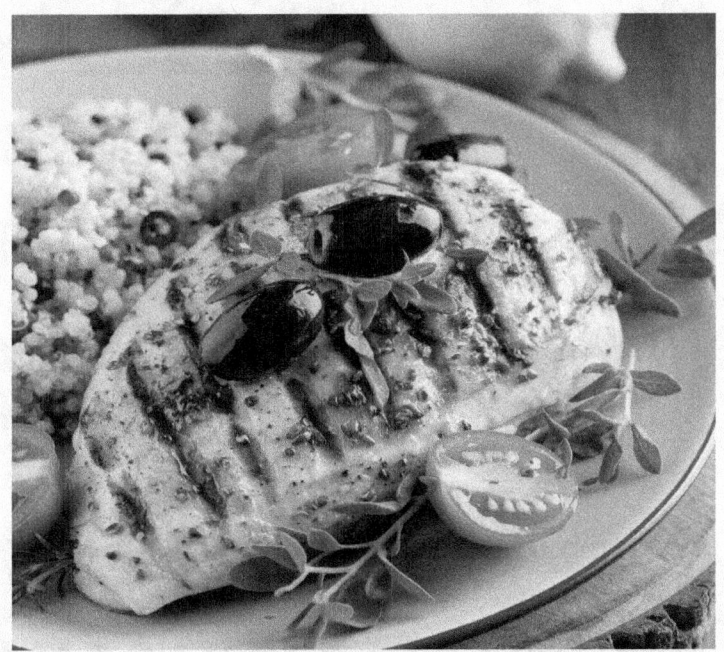

- 4 oz boneless, skinless chicken breast

  1 tablespoon olive oil

  Juice of 1/2 lemon

  1 teaspoon dried oregano

  Salt and pepper, to taste

  1 cup mixed salad greens

Preparation Method

- In a small bowl, mix olive oil, lemon juice, oregano, salt, and pepper. Marinate the chicken in this mixture for at least 15 minutes. Grill chicken over medium heat until cooked through, about 5-7 minutes per side. Serve over mixed greens.

Nutritional Value

- Calories: 210 kcal

  Protein: 25g

  Carbohydrates: 3g

  Fats: 8g

  GI: Low, with lean protein and fiber

Greek Yogurt with Walnuts and Berries

Ingredients

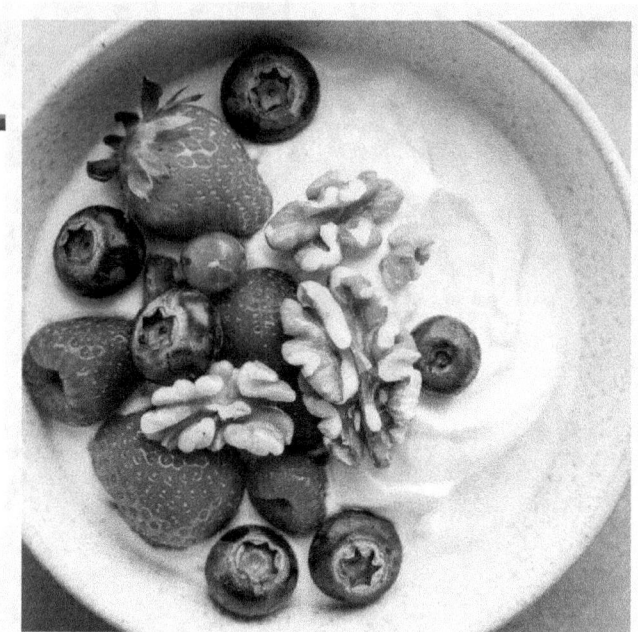

- 1 cup plain Greek yogurt

  1/4 cup mixed berries (blueberries, raspberries)

  1 tablespoon walnuts, chopped

  1/4 teaspoon cinnamon

Preparation Method

- Place Greek yogurt in a bowl, top with mixed berries and chopped walnuts, and sprinkle with

  cinnamon. Serve immediately.

Nutritional Value

- Calories: 180 kcal

  Protein: 12g

  Carbohydrates: 15g

  Fats: 8g

  GI: Low, with high protein and fiber

Quinoa Tabbouleh

Ingredients

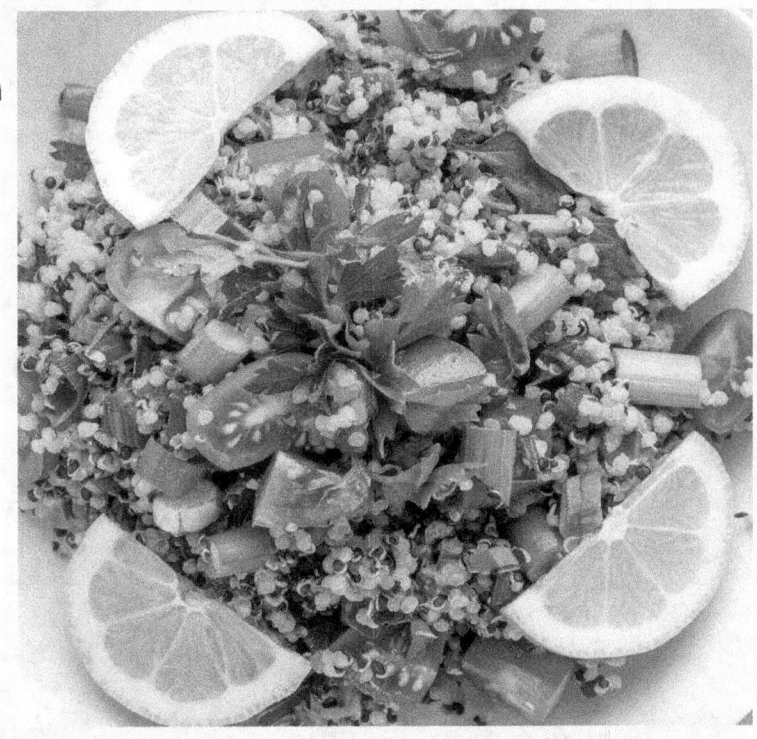

- 1/2 cup cooked quinoa

  1/4 cup diced cucumber

  1/4 cup cherry tomatoes, halved

  2 tablespoons fresh parsley, chopped

  1 tablespoon olive oil

  Juice of 1/2 lemon

  Salt and pepper, to taste

Preparation Method

- In a bowl, mix cooked quinoa with cucumber, tomatoes, and parsley. Drizzle with olive oil and lemon juice, then season with salt and pepper. Toss to combine and serve.

Nutritional Value

- Calories: 200 kcal

  Protein: 6g

  Carbohydrates: 25g (fiber-rich)

  Fats: 7g

  GI: Low, with complex carbs and healthy fats

Stuffed Bell Peppers with Lentils

● Ingredients

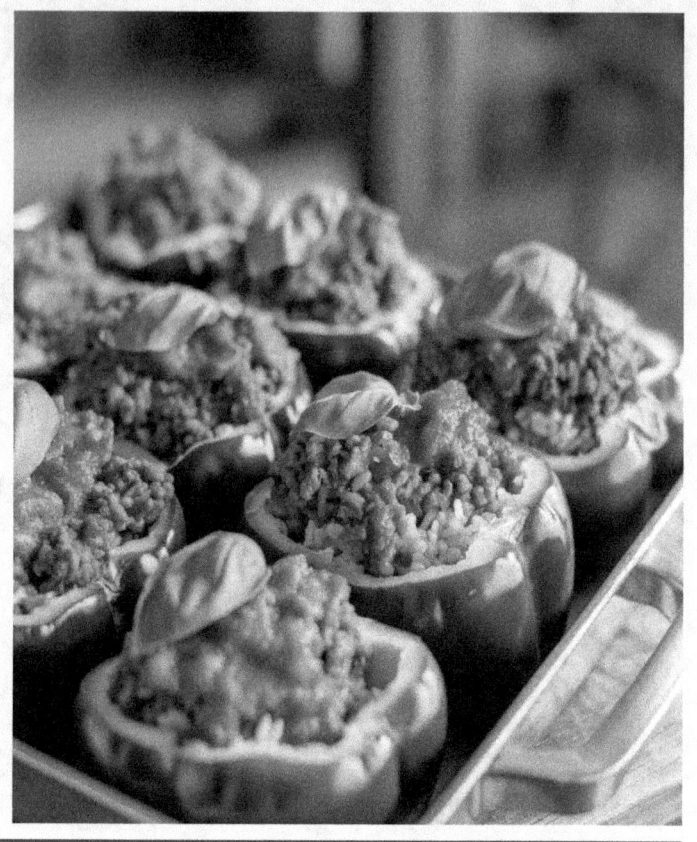

● 2 bell peppers, halved and seeds removed

1/2 cup cooked lentils

1/4 cup diced tomatoes

1/4 cup spinach, chopped

1 tablespoon olive oil

Salt and pepper, to taste

● Preparation Method

● Preheat oven to 375°F (190°C). Mix lentils, tomatoes, spinach, olive oil, salt, and pepper in a

bowl. Fill each pepper half with the mixture and bake for 20-25 minutes.

● Nutritional Value

● Calories: 210 kcal

Protein: 9g

Carbohydrates: 30g (fiber-rich)

Fats: 7g

GI: Low, with fiber-rich lentils

Zucchini Noodles with Pesto

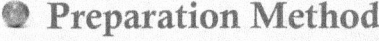 Ingredients

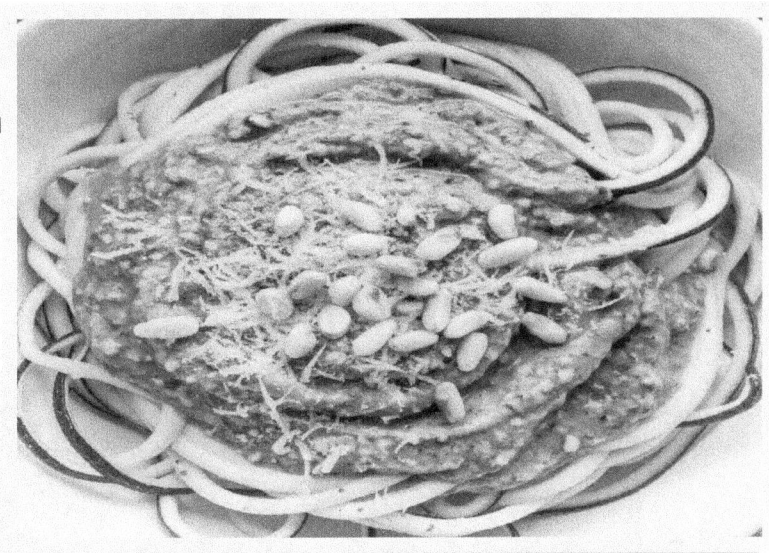

- 1 zucchini, spiralized

  2 tablespoons homemade pesto

  1/4 cup cherry tomatoes, halved

Preparation Method

- Lightly steam zucchini noodles for 2-3 minutes. Toss with pesto and garnish with cherry

  tomatoes.

Nutritional Value

- Calories: 150 kcal

  Protein: 4g

  Carbohydrates: 10g

  Fats: 8g

  GI: Low, with minimal carbs and healthy fats

Baked Cod with Olive Tapenade

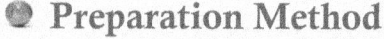 **Ingredients**

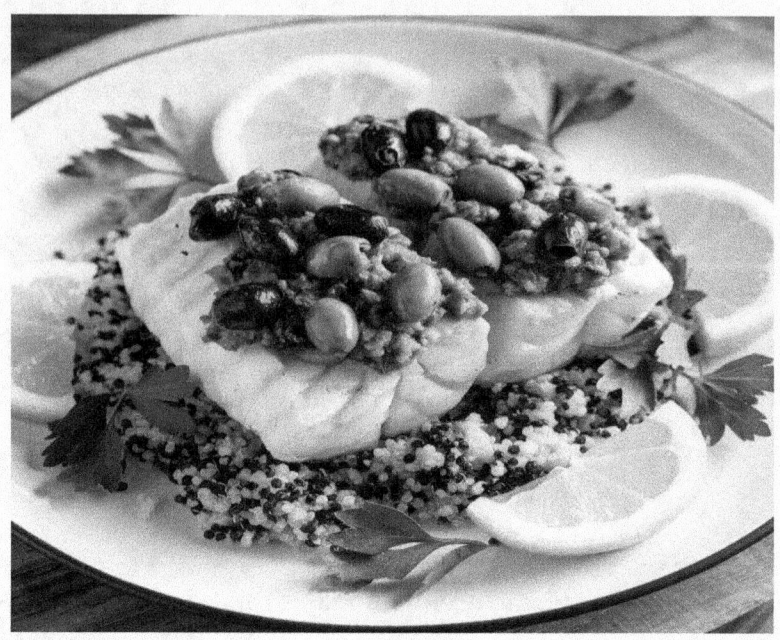

- 4 oz cod fillet

  1 tablespoon olive tapenade

  1/2 lemon, juiced

  1 cup steamed asparagus

Preparation Method

- Preheat oven to 400°F (200°C). Place cod fillet on a baking sheet, drizzle with lemon juice, and

  top with olive tapenade. Bake for 12-15 minutes. Serve with steamed asparagus.

Nutritional Value

- Calories: 210 kcal

  Protein: 22g

  Carbohydrates: 5g

  Fats: 8g

  GI: Low, with lean protein and fiber

Eggplant and Chickpea Stew

Ingredients

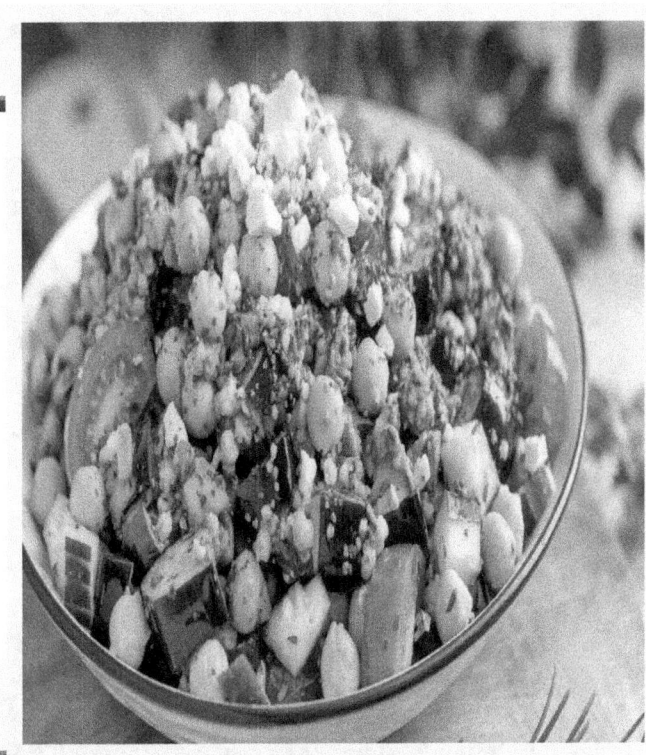

- 1/2 cup canned chickpeas, rinsed and drained

  1/2 eggplant, diced

  1 small onion, chopped

  1 garlic clove, minced

  1 tablespoon olive oil

  1/2 teaspoon cumin

  Salt and pepper, to taste

Preparation Method

- Heat olive oil in a pot, add onion and garlic, and sauté until soft. Add eggplant and cook until tender, then add chickpeas, cumin, salt, and pepper. Simmer for 10-15 minutes.

Nutritional Value

- Calories: 190 kcal

  Protein: 6g

  Carbohydrates: 25g (fiber-rich)

  Fats: 6g

  GI: Low, with fiber and healthy fats

Cauliflower and Tuna Salad

Ingredients

- 1/2 cup cauliflower florets, steamed

  1 can tuna in water, drained

  1 tablespoon olive oil

  Juice of half a lemon

  Salt and pepper, to taste

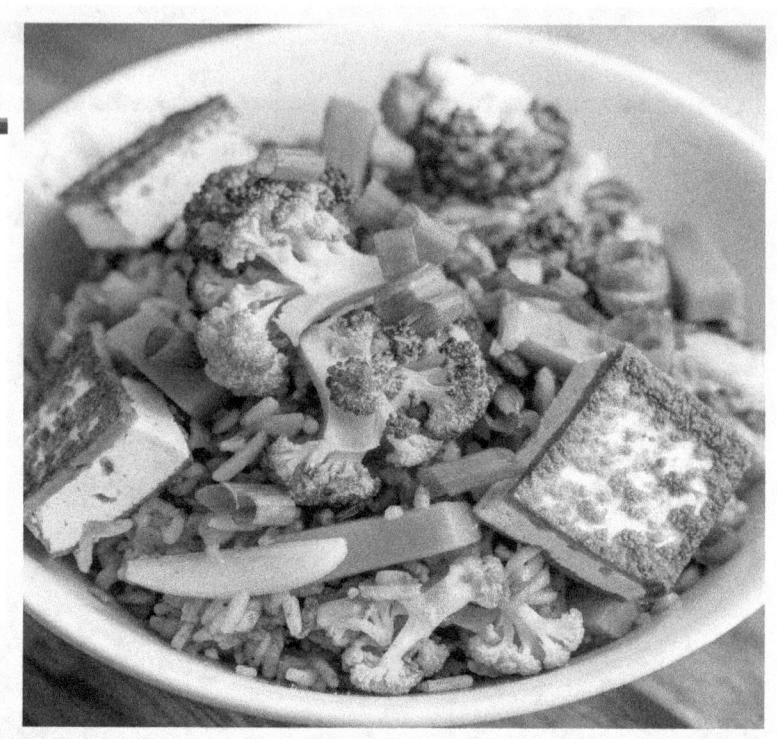

Preparation Method

- In a bowl, combine cauliflower and tuna. Drizzle with olive oil and lemon juice, season with salt and pepper, and toss to combine.

Nutritional Value

- Calories: 180 kcal

  Protein: 20g

  Carbohydrates: 5g

  Fats: 8g

  GI: Low, with high protein and fiber

Mediterranean Omelet

Ingredients

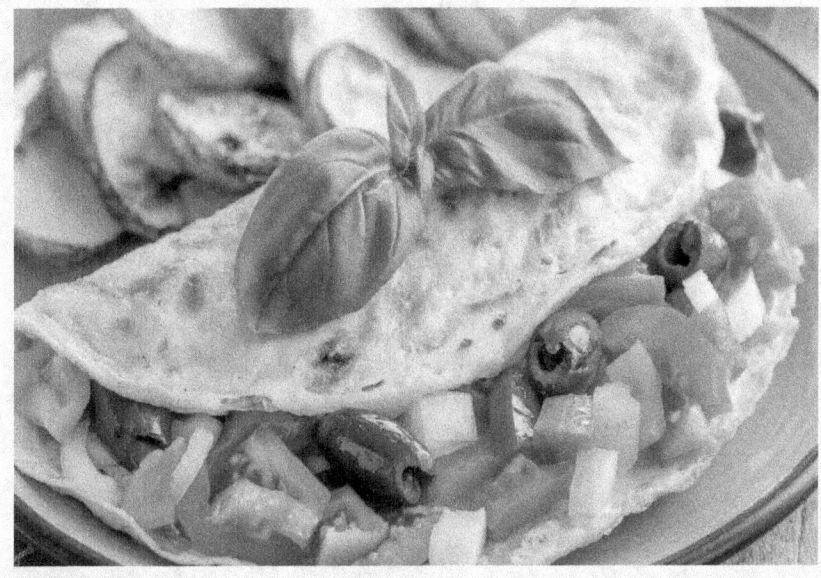

- 2 eggs or 1 egg + 2 egg whites

  1/4 cup diced tomatoes

  1/4 cup spinach, chopped

  1 tablespoon feta cheese

  Salt and pepper, to taste

Preparation Method

- Whisk eggs, add salt and pepper. Pour eggs into a heated skillet, add tomatoes and spinach, and cook until set. Sprinkle feta cheese before folding the omelet.

Nutritional Value

- Calories: 180 kcal

  Protein: 14g

  Carbohydrates: 4g

  Fats: 10g

  GI: Low, with high protein

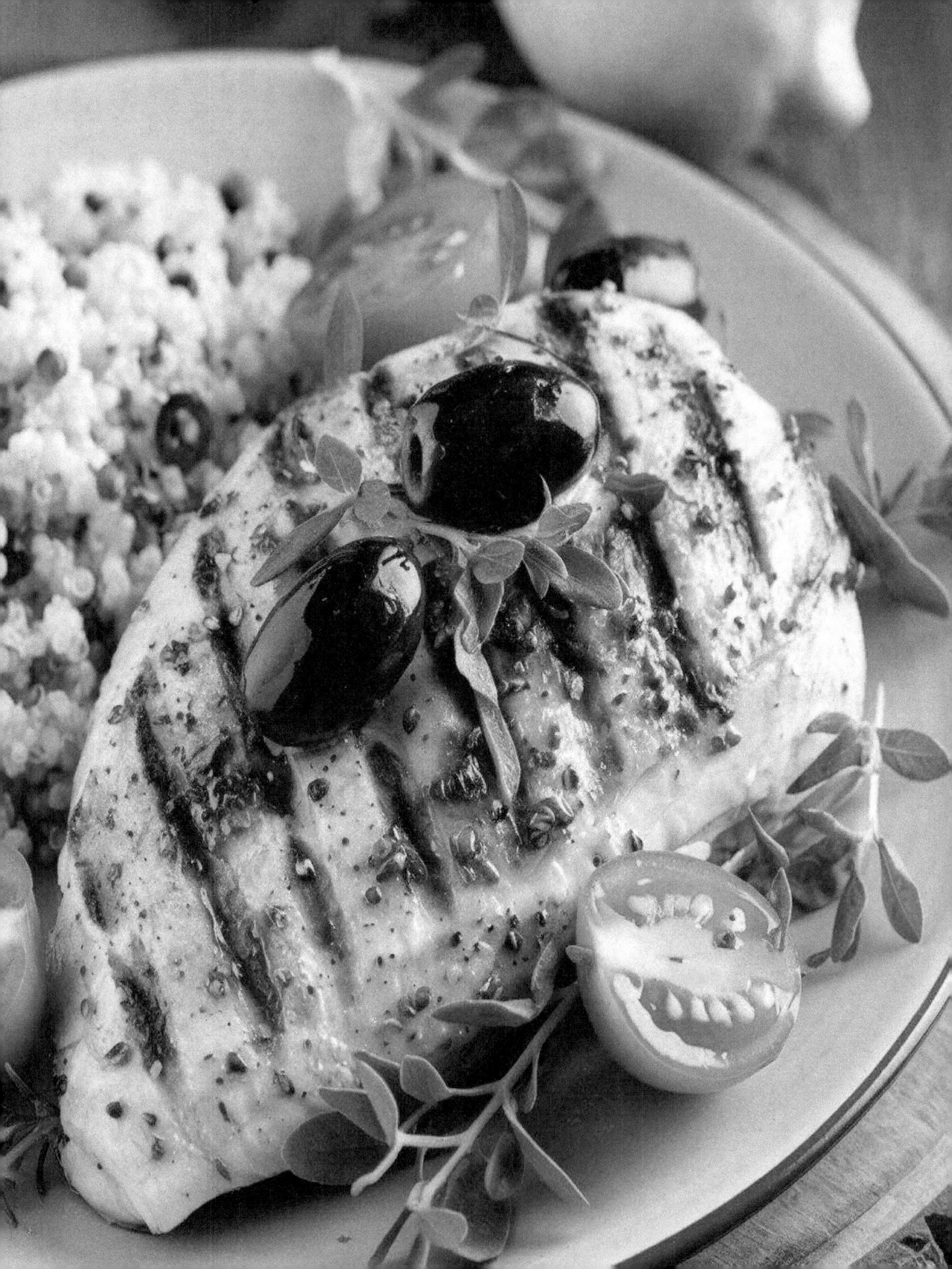

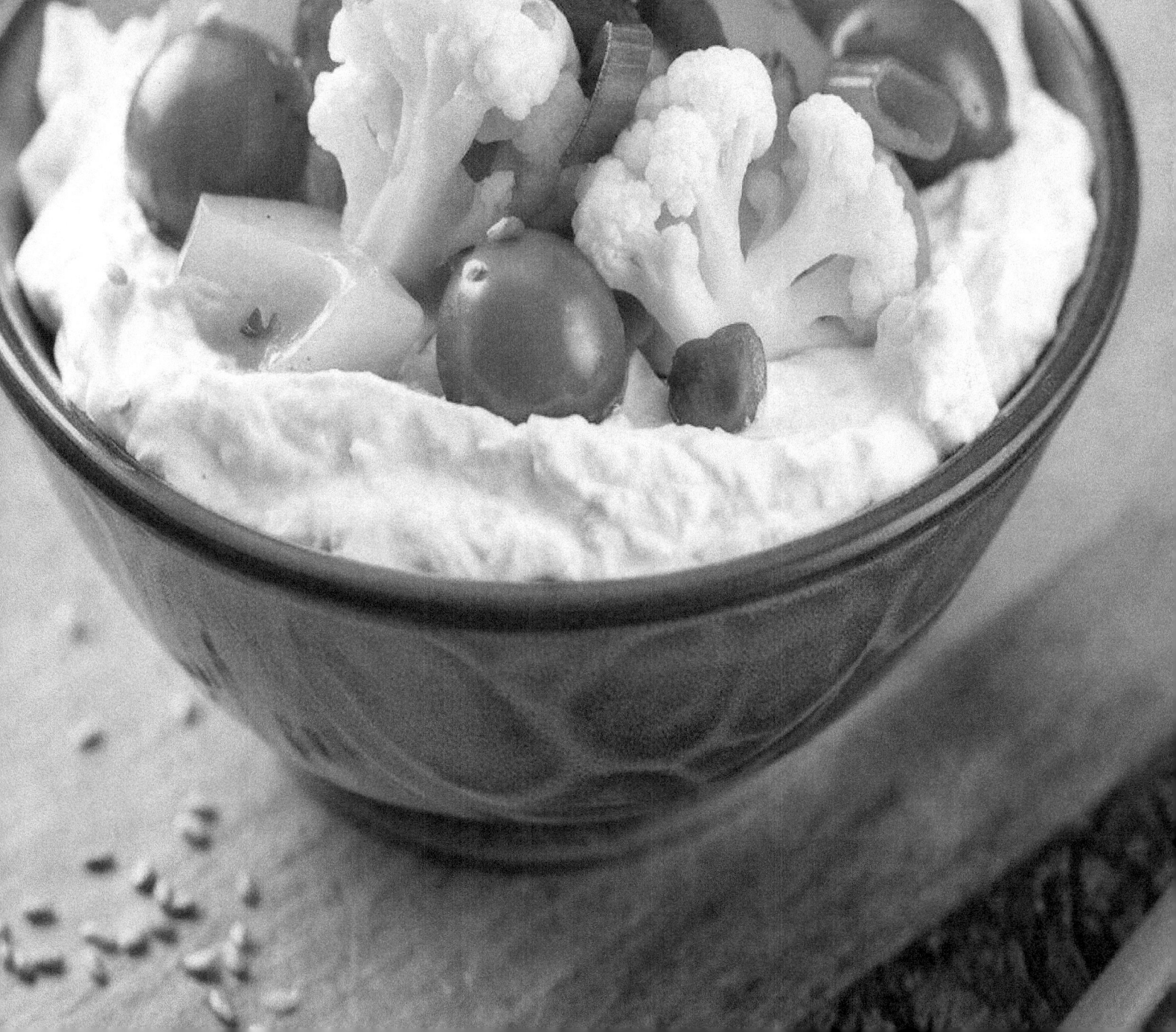

PLANT BASED DIET

RECIPES

Lentil and Spinach Stew

Ingredients

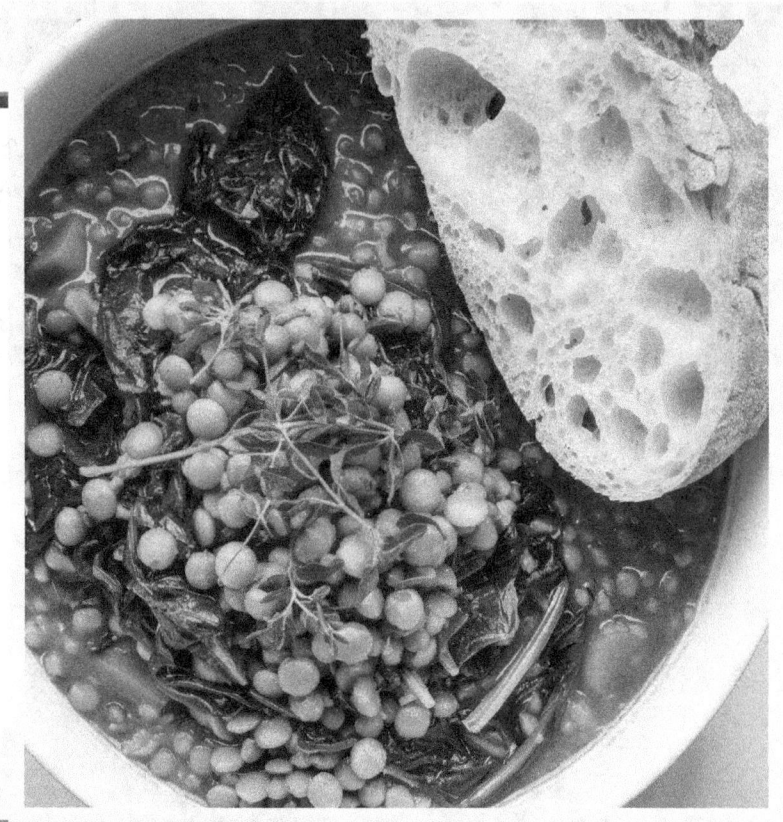

- 1 cup green or brown lentils, rinsed

  2 cups spinach, chopped

  1 carrot, diced

  1 onion, chopped

  2 cloves garlic, minced

  1 tablespoon olive oil

  4 cups vegetable broth

  Salt and pepper, to taste

Preparation Method

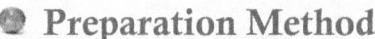

- In a large pot, heat olive oil and sauté the onion, garlic, and carrot until soft. Add lentils and vegetable broth, bring to a boil, then reduce heat and simmer for 20-25 minutes. Stir in spinach, cook for 5 more minutes, and season with salt and pepper.

Nutritional Value

- Calories: 250 kcal

  Protein: 15g

  Carbohydrates: 40g (fiber-rich)

  Fats: 4g

  GI: Low, with fiber and plant protein

Chickpea and Vegetable Stir-Fry

● Ingredients

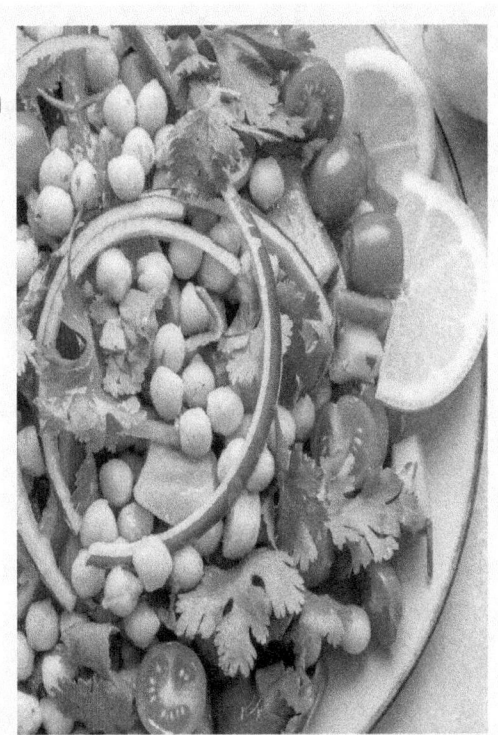

● 1 cup canned chickpeas, rinsed and drained

1/2 bell pepper, sliced

1/2 zucchini, sliced

1/2 cup broccoli florets

2 tablespoons coconut aminos or low-sodium soy sauce

1 tablespoon olive oil

1 clove garlic, minced

● Preparation Method

● Heat olive oil in a skillet, add garlic, and sauté for 1 minute. Add vegetables and stir-fry until tender-crisp. Add chickpeas and coconut aminos, then cook for another 3-4 minutes.

● Nutritional Value

● Calories: 220 kcal

Protein: 9g

Carbohydrates: 28g (fiber-rich)

Fats: 8g

GI: Low, with fiber and healthy fats

Quinoa Salad with Avocado and Black Beans

Ingredients

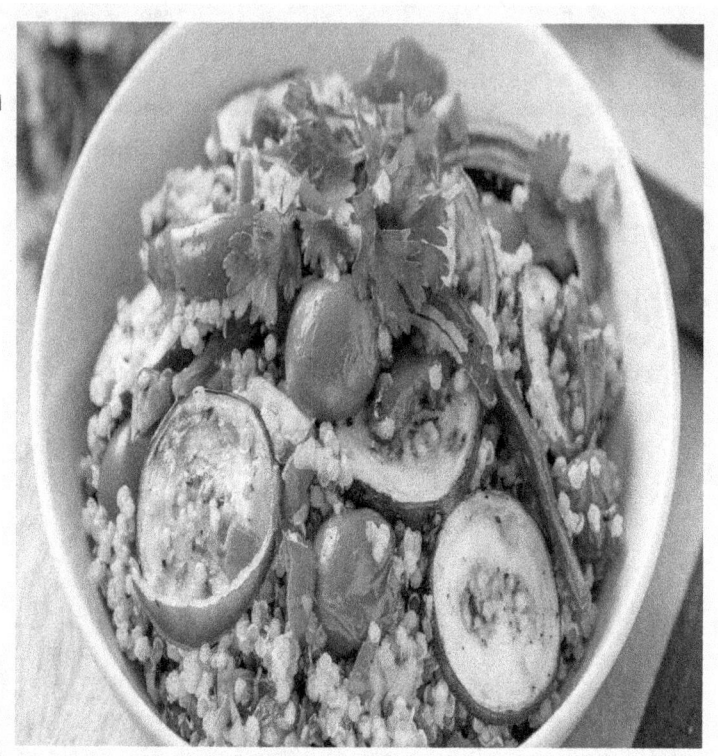

- 1/2 cup cooked quinoa

  1/4 cup black beans, rinsed and drained

  1/4 avocado, diced

  1/4 cup cherry tomatoes, halved

  1 tablespoon olive oil

  Juice of half a lime

  Salt and pepper, to taste

Preparation Method

- In a bowl, mix quinoa, black beans, avocado, and tomatoes. Drizzle with olive oil and lime juice, season with salt and pepper, and toss well.

Nutritional Value

- Calories: 270 kcal

  Protein: 9g

  Carbohydrates: 30g

  Fats: 12g

  GI: Low, with fiber and healthy fats

Cauliflower and Sweet Potato Curry

● Ingredients

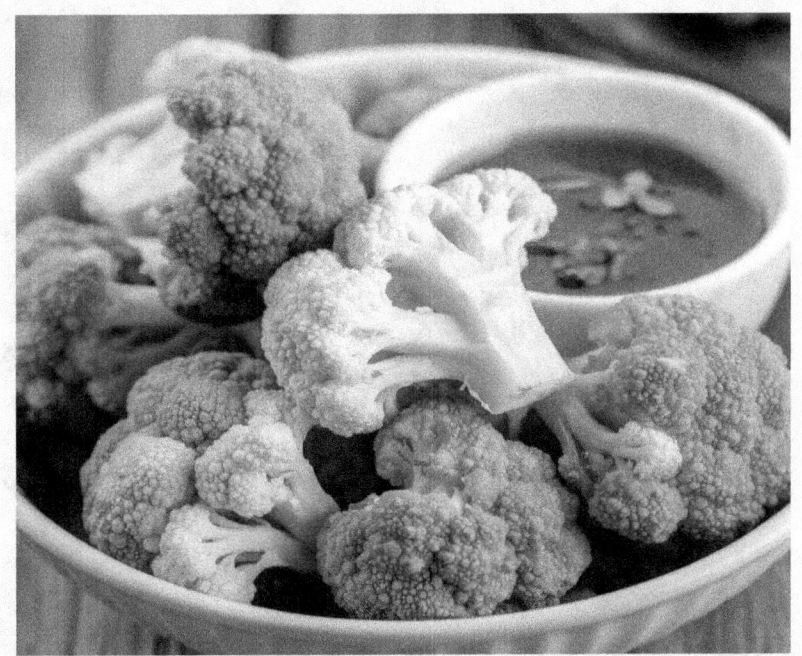

- ● 1/2 cup cauliflower florets

  1/2 cup diced sweet potato

  1/4 cup coconut milk

  1/2 cup vegetable broth

  1 teaspoon curry powder

  Salt, to taste

● Preparation Method

● In a pot, combine vegetable broth, coconut milk, curry powder, cauliflower, and sweet potato.

Simmer for 15-20 minutes until the vegetables are tender. Season with salt.

● Nutritional Value

● Calories: 210 kcal

Protein: 4g

Carbohydrates: 30g

Fats: 10g

GI: Low, with complex carbs and fiber

Stuffed Bell Peppers with Brown Rice and Vegetables

Ingredients

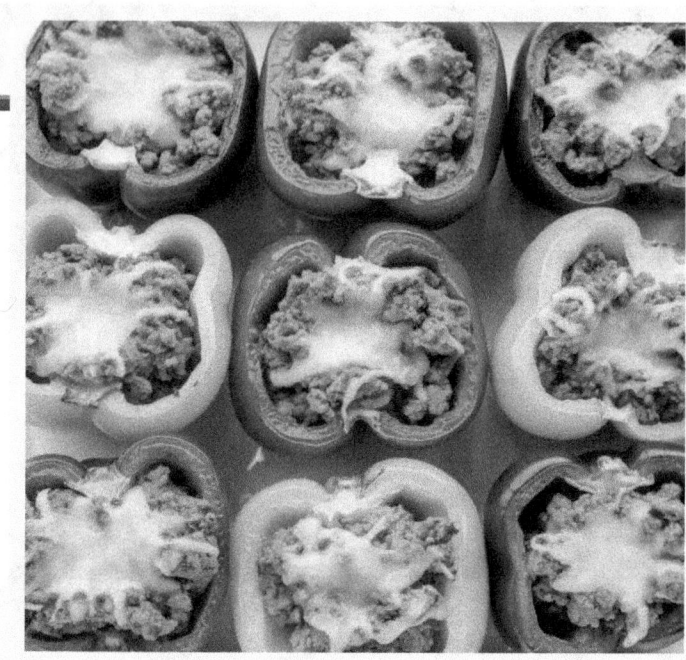

- 1 bell pepper, halved and seeds removed

  1/2 cup cooked brown rice

  1/4 cup diced tomatoes

  1/4 cup mushrooms, diced

  1 tablespoon olive oil

  Salt and pepper, to taste

Preparation Method

- Preheat oven to 375°F (190°C). In a bowl, mix rice, tomatoes, mushrooms, and olive oil. Stuff the bell pepper halves with the mixture, place in a baking dish, and bake for 20-25 minutes.

Nutritional Value

- Calories: 240 kcal

  Protein: 5g

  Carbohydrates: 40g (fiber-rich)

  Fats: 8g

  GI: Low, with fiber-rich grains and vegetables

Zucchini Noodles with Tomato Basil Sauce

Ingredients

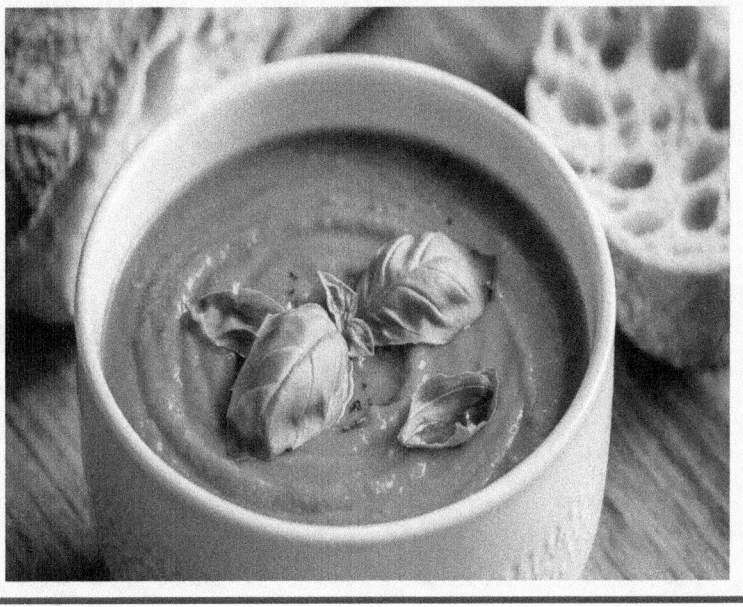

- 1 zucchini, spiralized

  1/2 cup cherry tomatoes, halved

  1 tablespoon olive oil

  2 tablespoons fresh basil, chopped

  Salt and pepper, to taste

Preparation Method

- In a skillet, heat olive oil, add cherry tomatoes, and cook until soft. Toss zucchini noodles with

  the tomato sauce and garnish with fresh basil.

Nutritional Value

- Calories: 130 kcal

  Protein: 3g

  Carbohydrates: 10g

  Fats: 8g

  GI: Low, with minimal carbs and healthy fats

Roasted Vegetable and Hummus Wrap

◉ Ingredients

◉ 1 whole-grain wrap

1/4 cup hummus

1/4 cup roasted vegetables (bell pepper, zucchini, eggplant)

Handful of arugula

◉ Preparation Method

◉ Spread hummus on the wrap, layer with roasted vegetables and arugula, and roll tightly. Serve fresh.

◉ Nutritional Value

◉ Calories: 230 kcal

Protein: 7g

Carbohydrates: 35g

Fats: 7g

GI: Low, with fiber-rich grains and healthy fats

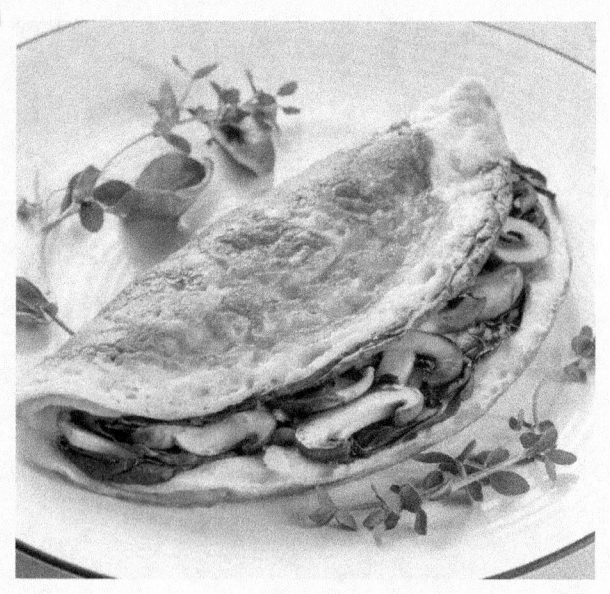

Mediterranean Lentil Salad

Ingredients

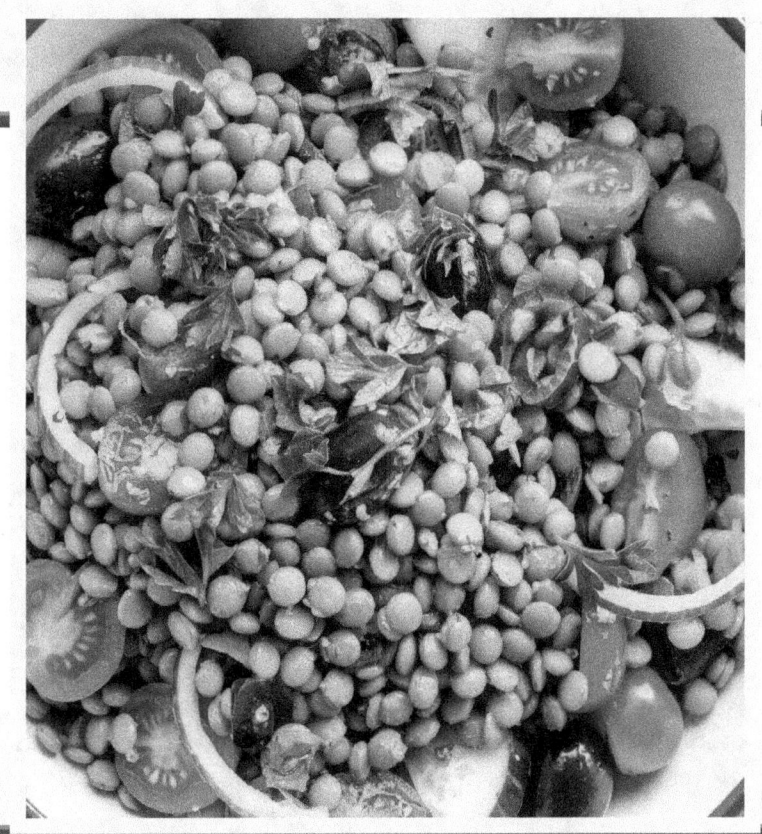

- 1/2 cup cooked lentils

  1/4 cup cucumber, diced

  1/4 cup cherry tomatoes, halved

  1 tablespoon olive oil

  Juice of half a lemon

  Salt and pepper, to taste

Preparation Method

- In a bowl, mix lentils, cucumber, and tomatoes. Drizzle with olive oil and lemon juice, season

  with salt and pepper, and toss well.

Nutritional Value

- Calories: 200 kcal

  Protein: 9g

  Carbohydrates: 30g

  Fats: 7g

  GI: Low, with high fiber

Tofu Stir-Fry with Broccoli and Snap Peas

Ingredients

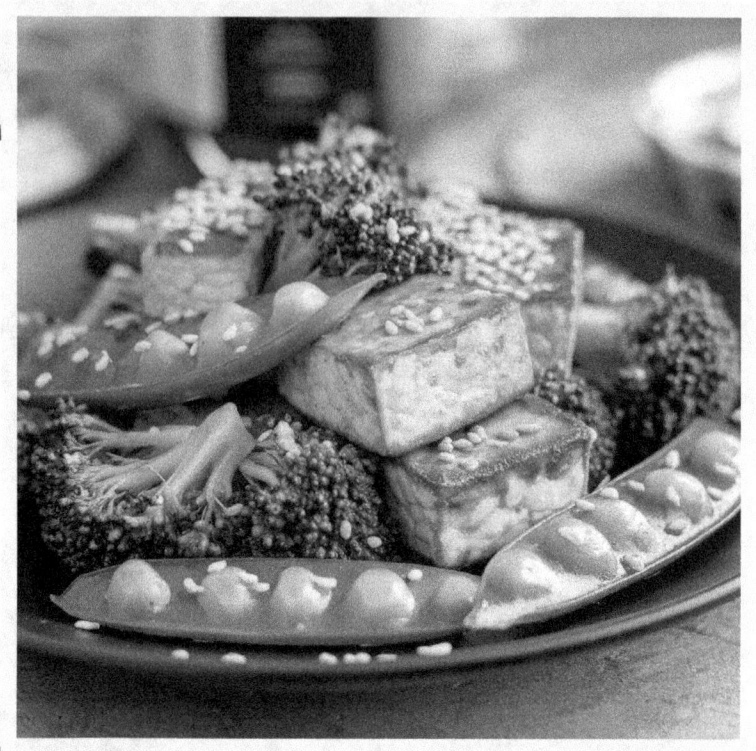

- 4 oz tofu, cubed

  1/2 cup broccoli florets

  1/4 cup snap peas

  1 tablespoon olive oil

  1 tablespoon coconut aminos

Preparation Method

- Heat olive oil in a skillet, add tofu, and cook until lightly browned. Add broccoli, snap peas, and

  coconut aminos, then stir-fry for 3-4 minutes until tender.

Nutritional Value

- Calories: 190 kcal

  Protein: 10g

  Carbohydrates: 12g

  Fats: 10g

  GI: Low, with plant protein and fiber

Baked Falafel with Cucumber Salad

Ingredients

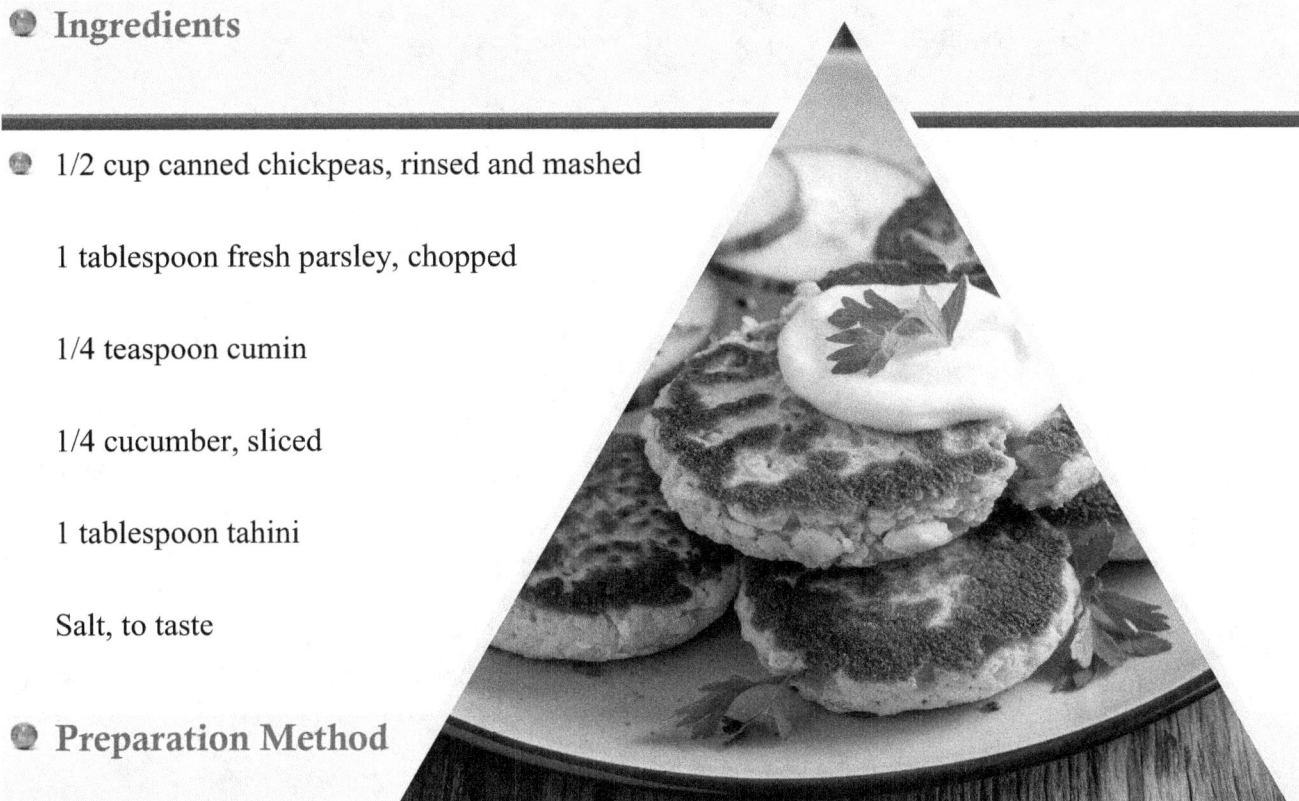

- 1/2 cup canned chickpeas, rinsed and mashed

  1 tablespoon fresh parsley, chopped

  1/4 teaspoon cumin

  1/4 cucumber, sliced

  1 tablespoon tahini

  Salt, to taste

Preparation Method

- Preheat oven to 375°F (190°C). Mix chickpeas, parsley, cumin, and salt, form into small patties, and bake for 15-20 minutes. Serve with cucumber slices and a drizzle of tahini.

Nutritional Value

- Calories: 200 kcal

  Protein: 8g

  Carbohydrates: 25g

  Fats: 8g

  GI: Low, with high fiber and healthy fats

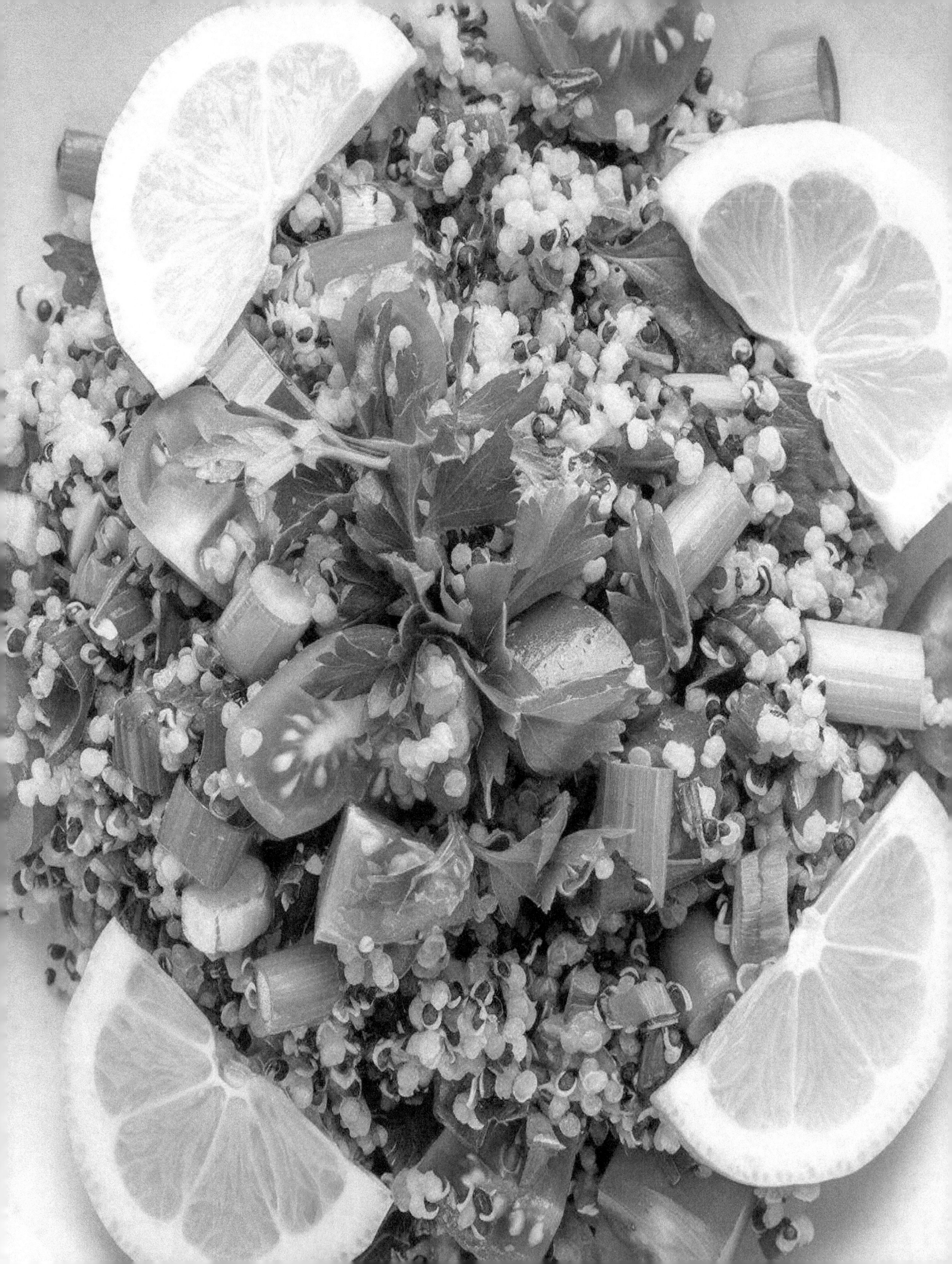

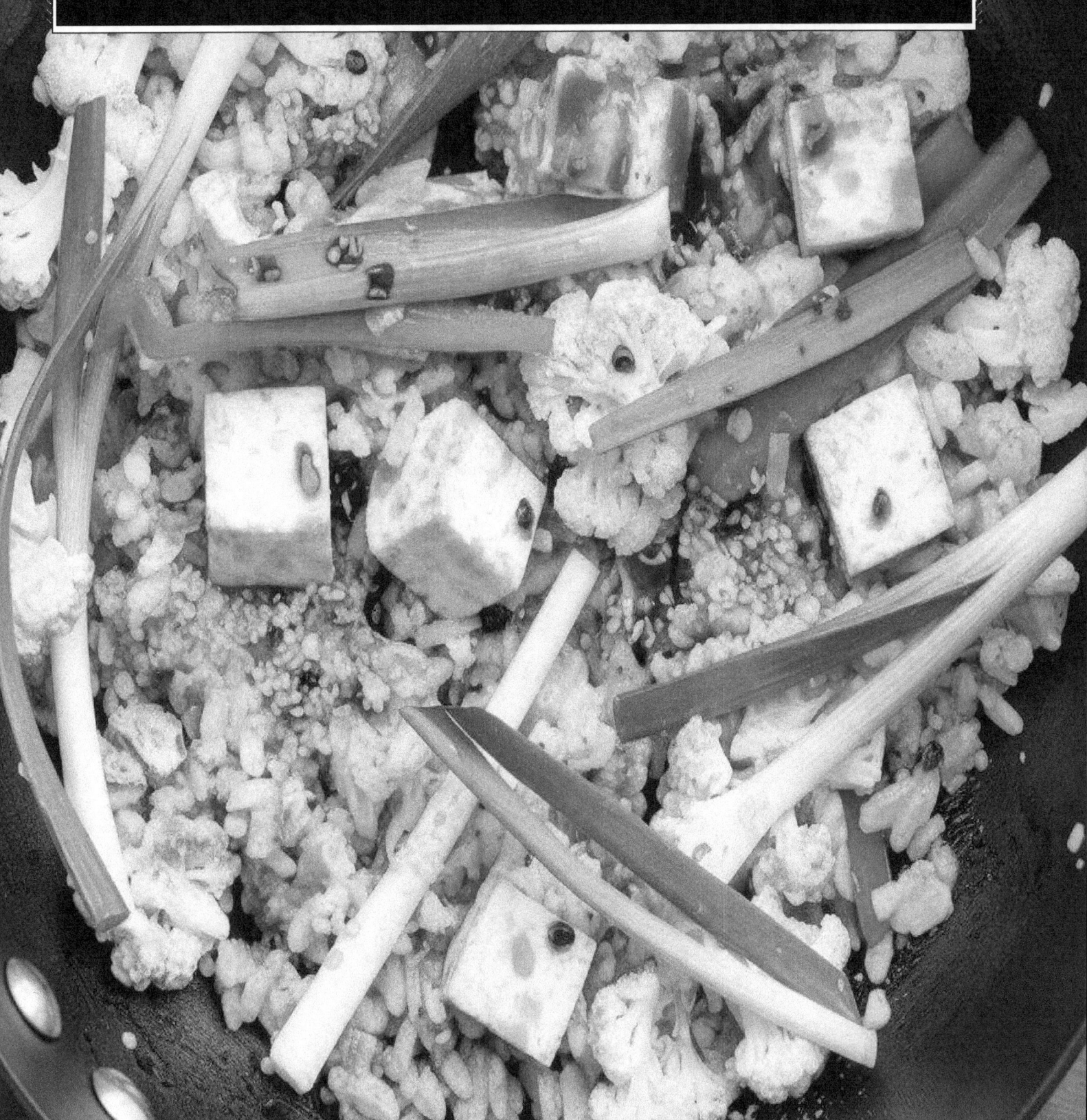

DASH DIET RECIPES

Berry and Oatmeal Bowl

Ingredients

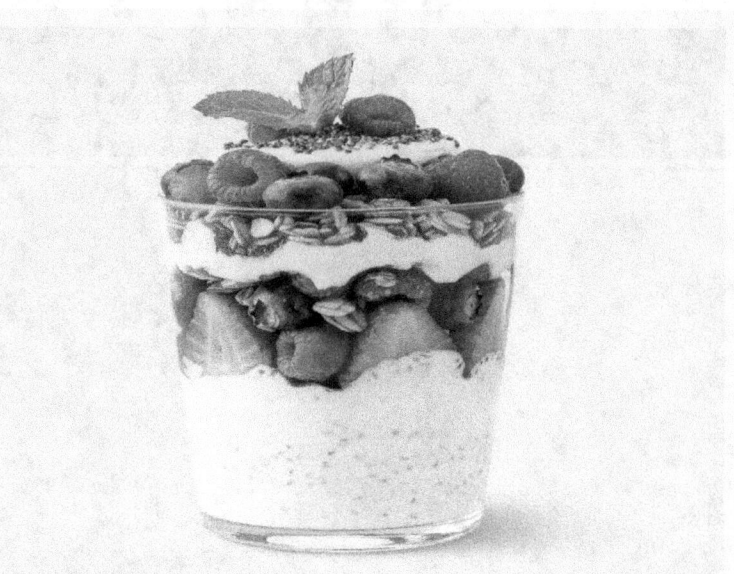

- 1/2 cup rolled oats

  1 cup unsweetened almond milk

  1/4 cup blueberries

  1/4 cup raspberries

  1 tablespoon chia seeds

Preparation Method

- In a saucepan, combine oats and almond milk and cook over medium heat until thickened. Top with blueberries, raspberries, and chia seeds.

Nutritional Value

- Calories: 210 kcal

  Protein: 6g

  Carbohydrates: 38g

  Fats: 5g

  Fiber: 9g

  GI: Low, with fiber-rich berries and whole grains

Spinach and Mushroom Egg White Scramble

Ingredients

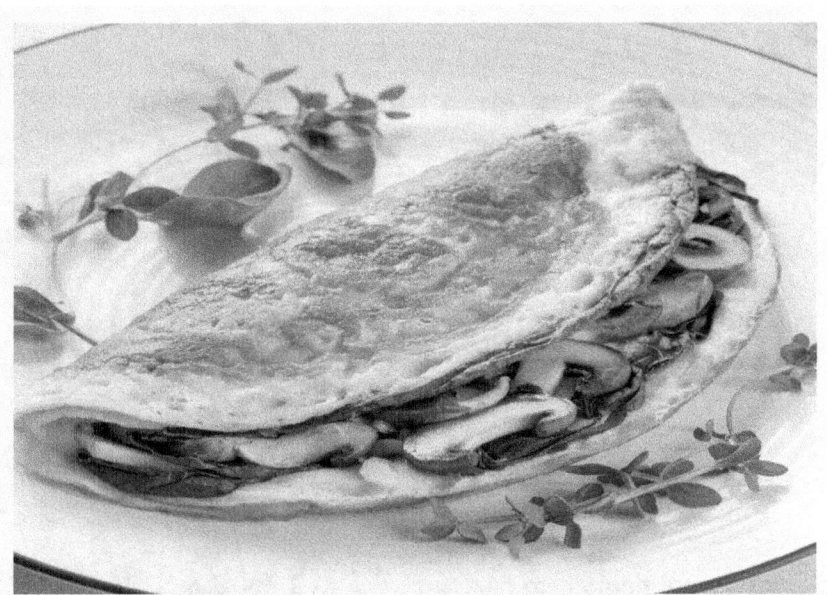

- 4 egg whites

  1 cup spinach, chopped

  1/2 cup mushrooms, sliced

  1 tablespoon olive oil

  Salt and pepper, to taste

Preparation Method

- Heat olive oil in a skillet, add mushrooms, and cook until softened. Add spinach and egg whites, stirring until eggs are set. Season with salt and pepper.

Nutritional Value

- Calories: 140 kcal

  Protein: 15g

  Carbohydrates: 4g

  Fats: 7g

  GI: Low, with high protein and fiber

Quinoa and Black Bean Salad

Ingredients

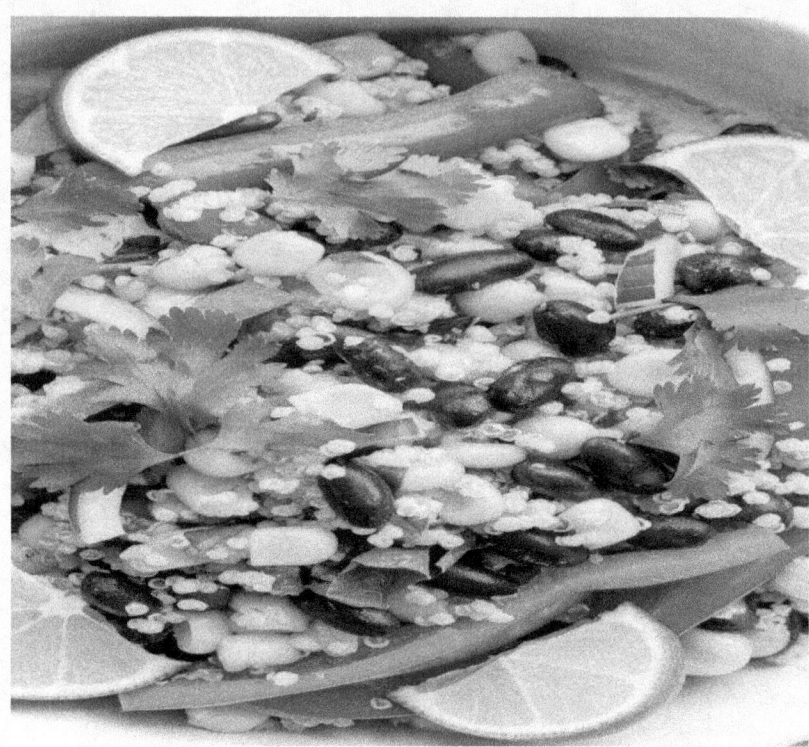

- 1/2 cup cooked quinoa

  1/4 cup black beans, rinsed

  1/4 cup diced cucumber

  1/4 cup diced tomatoes

  1 tablespoon olive oil

  Juice of half a lime

  Salt and pepper, to taste

Preparation Method

- Combine quinoa, black beans, cucumber, and tomatoes in a bowl. Drizzle with olive oil and lime juice, then toss to mix. Season with salt and pepper.

Nutritional Value

- Calories: 220 kcal

  Protein: 7g

  Carbohydrates: 36g

  Fats: 8g

  GI: Low, with high fiber and plant-based protein

Greek Yogurt with Nuts and Berries

Ingredients

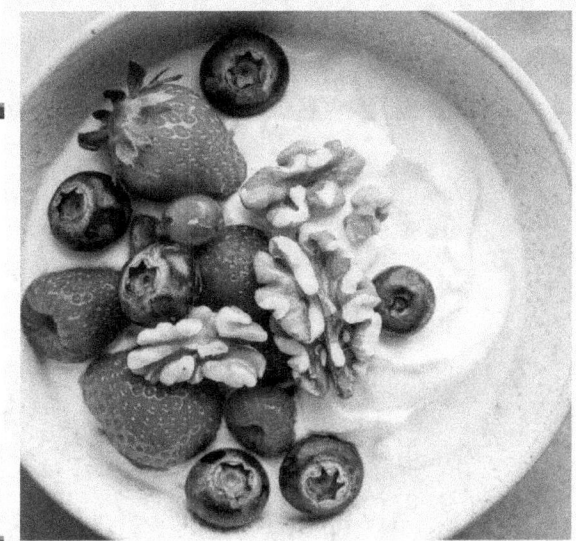

- 1/2 cup plain Greek yogurt

  1 tablespoon almonds, chopped

  1 tablespoon walnuts, chopped

  1/4 cup mixed berries (blueberries and strawberries)

Preparation Method

- Top Greek yogurt with berries, almonds, and walnuts for a quick, protein-packed breakfast or snack.

Nutritional Value

- Calories: 180 kcal

  Protein: 12g

  Carbohydrates: 15g

  Fats: 8g

  GI: Low, with healthy fats and probiotics

Lemon Garlic Salmon with Asparagus

Ingredients

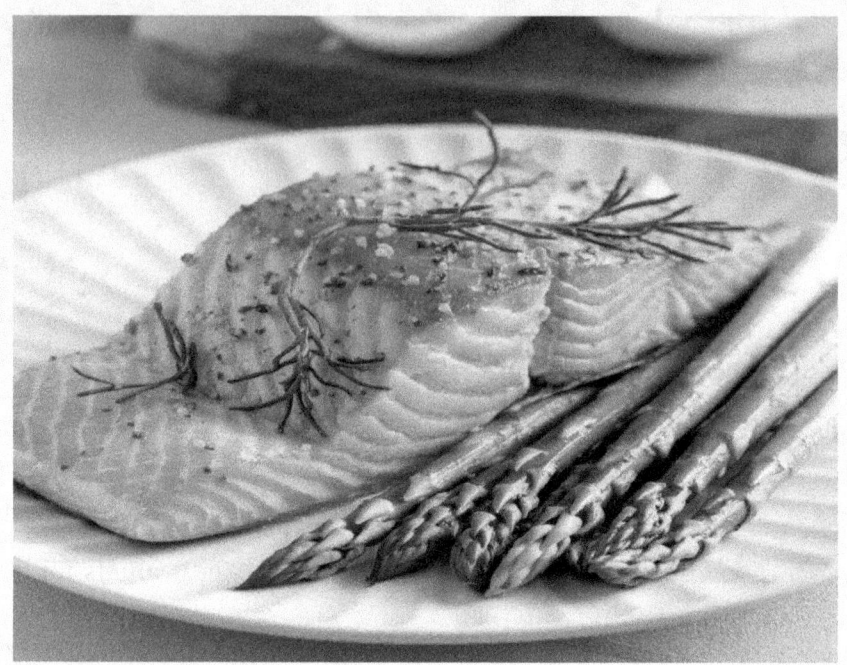

- 4 oz salmon fillet

  1 cup asparagus, trimmed

  1 teaspoon olive oil

  1 clove garlic, minced

  Juice of half a lemon

  Salt and pepper, to taste

Preparation Method

- Preheat oven to 400°F (200°C). Place salmon on a baking sheet with asparagus, drizzle with olive oil and lemon juice, then sprinkle garlic, salt, and pepper. Bake for 15 minutes until salmon flakes easily.

Nutritional Value

- Calories: 250 kcal

  Protein: 23g

  Carbohydrates: 5g

  Fats: 15g

  GI: Low, with lean protein and healthy fats

Chickpea and Cucumber Salad

Ingredients

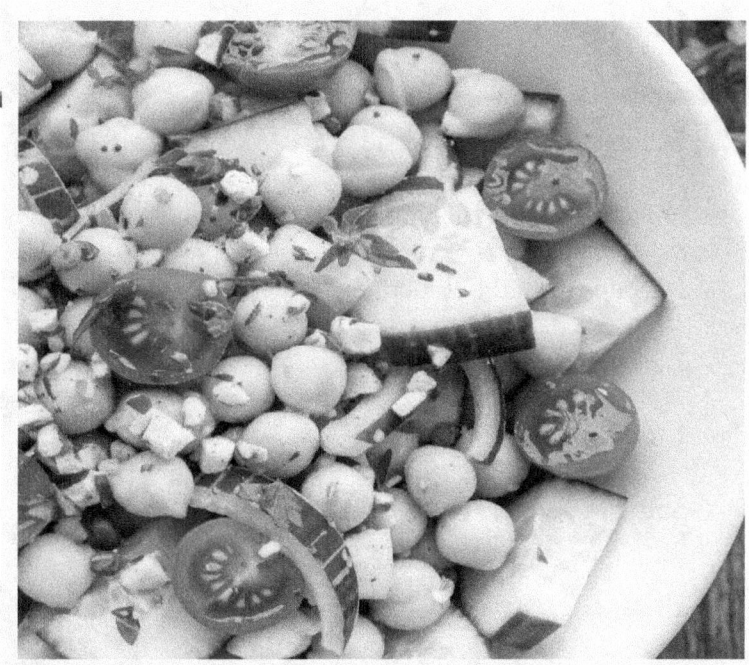

- 1/2 cup canned chickpeas, rinsed

  1/4 cup cucumber, diced

  1/4 cup cherry tomatoes, halved

  1 tablespoon olive oil

  1 tablespoon fresh parsley, chopped

  Salt and pepper, to taste

Preparation Method

- In a bowl, combine chickpeas, cucumber, tomatoes, and parsley. Drizzle with olive oil, season with salt and pepper, and mix well.

Nutritional Value

- Calories: 180 kcal

  Protein: 6g

  Carbohydrates: 22g

  Fats: 8g

  GI: Low, with fiber-rich legumes and vegetables

Roasted Veggie and Brown Rice Bowl

Ingredients

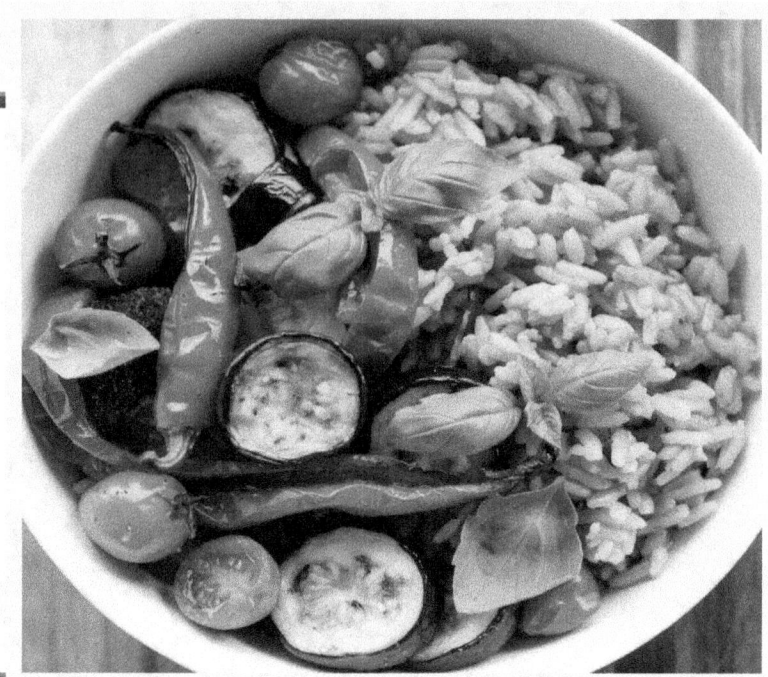

- 1/2 cup cooked brown rice

  1/2 cup roasted zucchini

  1/2 cup roasted bell pepper

  1/2 cup roasted cauliflower

  1 tablespoon olive oil

  Salt and pepper, to taste

Preparation Method

- Preheat oven to 400°F (200°C). Toss vegetables with olive oil, salt, and pepper, and roast for 20 minutes. Serve over brown rice.

Nutritional Value

- Calories: 300 kcal

  Protein: 8g

  Carbohydrates: 45g

  Fats: 10g

  GI: Low, with fiber-rich whole grains and vegetables

Mixed Bean Soup

Ingredients

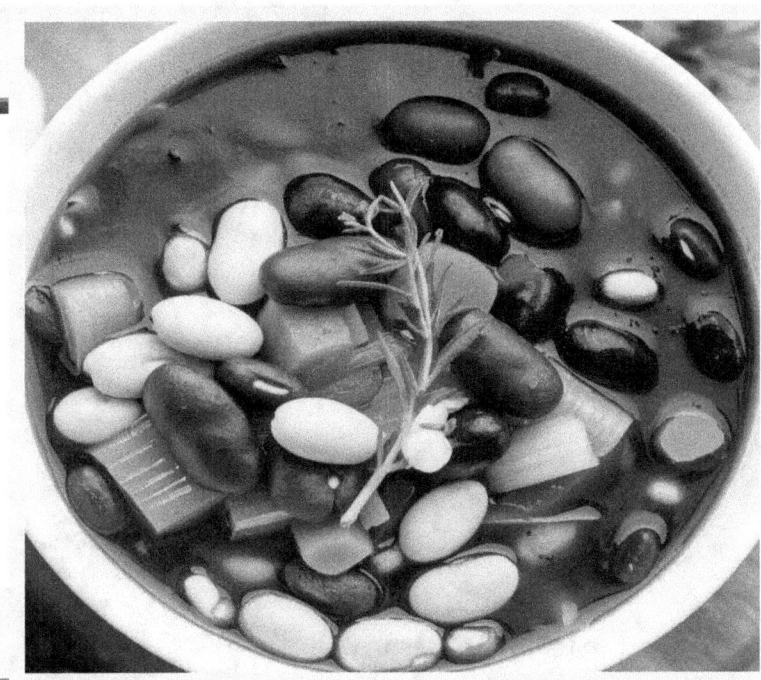

- 1/4 cup canned black beans, rinsed

  1/4 cup canned kidney beans, rinsed

  1/4 cup diced carrots

  1/4 cup diced celery

  1/2 cup vegetable broth

  Salt and pepper, to taste

Preparation Method

- Combine beans, carrots, celery, and broth in a pot. Simmer for 15-20 minutes until vegetables are tender. Season with salt and pepper.

Nutritional Value

- Calories: 150 kcal

  Protein: 9g

  Carbohydrates: 24g

  Fats: 1g

  GI: Low, with high fiber and plant-based protein

Baked Sweet Potato with Black Beans and Avocado

Ingredients

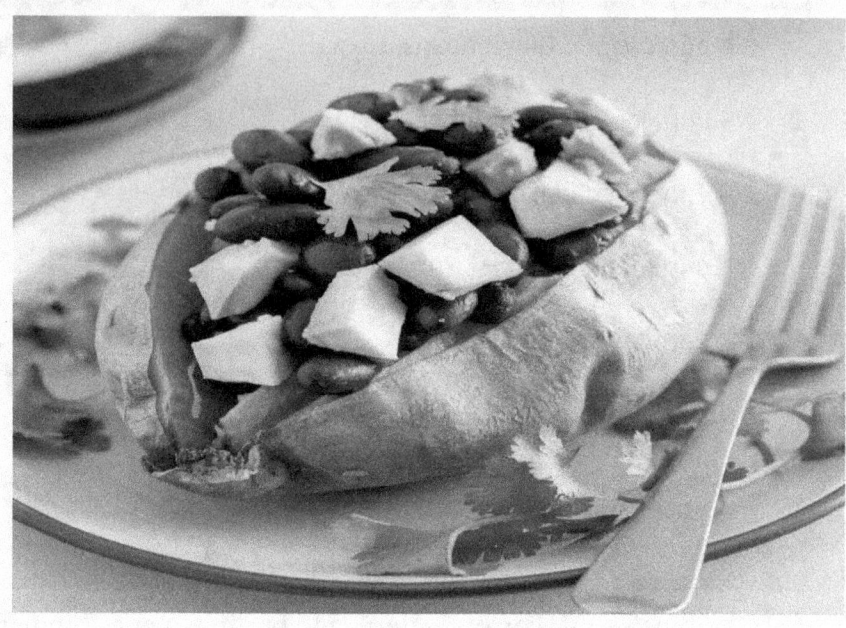

- 1 medium sweet potato

  1/4 cup black beans, rinsed

  1/4 avocado, diced

  1 tablespoon Greek yogurt

  Salt and pepper, to taste

Preparation Method

- Bake sweet potato at 400°F (200°C) for 40 minutes until tender. Top with black beans, avocado, and a dollop of Greek yogurt.

Nutritional Value

- Calories: 260 kcal

  Protein: 6g

  Carbohydrates: 40g

  Fats: 9g

  GI: Moderate, with complex carbs and fiber

Farro Salad with Tomatoes and Basil

Ingredients

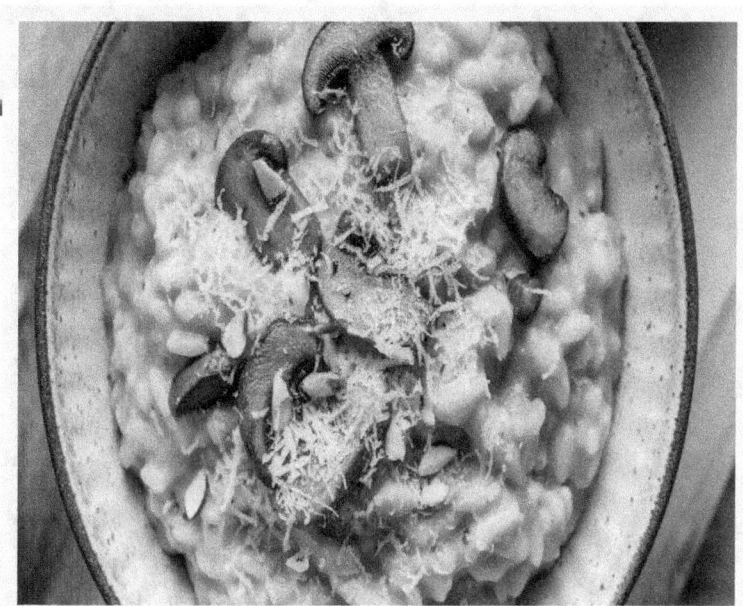

- 1/2 cup cooked farro

  1/4 cup cherry tomatoes, halved

  1 tablespoon fresh basil, chopped

  1 tablespoon olive oil

  Salt and pepper, to taste

Preparation Method

- Combine farro, tomatoes, and basil in a bowl. Drizzle with olive oil, season with salt and pepper, and toss well.

Nutritional Value

- Calories: 210 kcal

  Protein: 5g

  Carbohydrates: 34g

  Fats: 7g

  GI: Low, with fiber-rich ancient grains

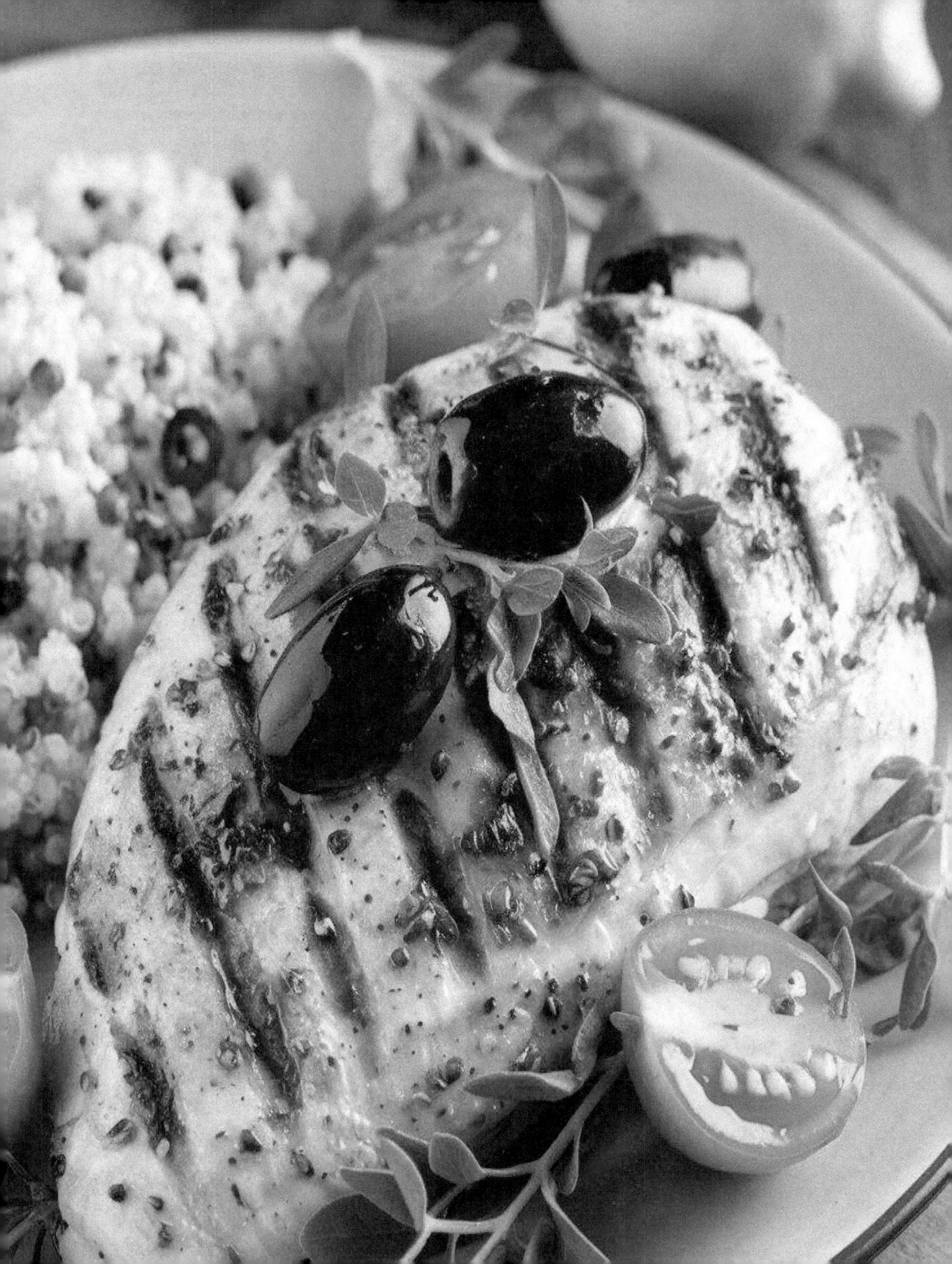

ANTI-INFLAMMATORY DIET FOR PREDIABETES

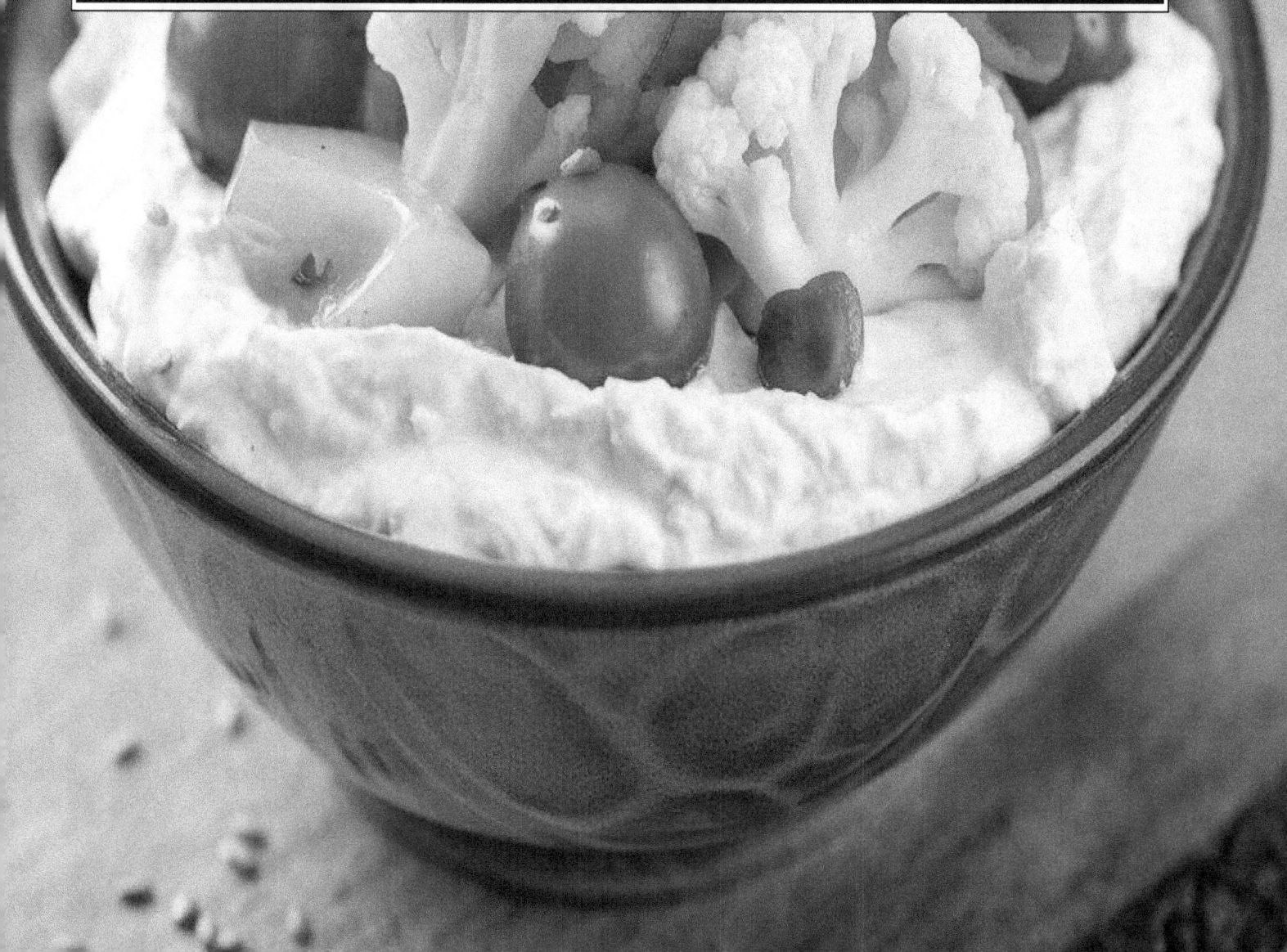

Turmeric Quinoa with Roasted Vegetables

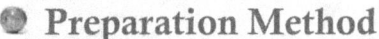 **Ingredients**

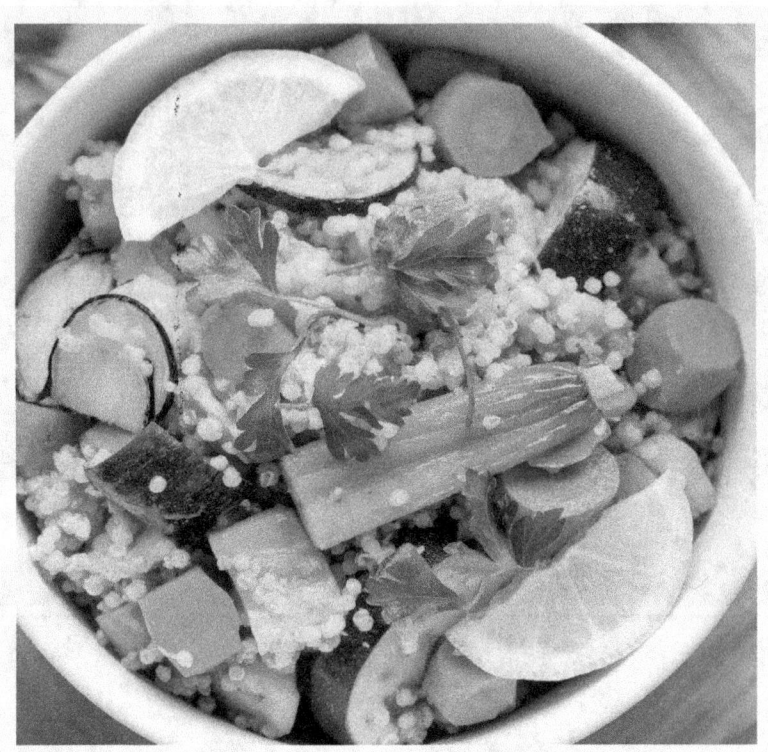

- 1/2 cup quinoa, rinsed

  1 cup water

  1/2 teaspoon turmeric

  1/4 teaspoon black pepper

  1/2 cup roasted broccoli

  1/2 cup roasted bell pepper

  1 tablespoon olive oil

Preparation Method

Cook quinoa in water with turmeric and black pepper until water is absorbed. Combine with roasted vegetables and drizzle with olive oil before serving.

Nutritional Value

Calories: 210 kcal

Protein: 8g

Carbohydrates: 34g

Fats: 8g

Fiber: 7g

Anti-inflammatory components: Turmeric, black pepper, vegetables, and whole grains

Spinach and Berry Smoothie

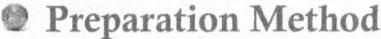 Ingredients

- 1 cup spinach

  1/2 cup blueberries

  1/2 cup strawberries

  1/2 cup unsweetened almond milk

  1 tablespoon chia seeds

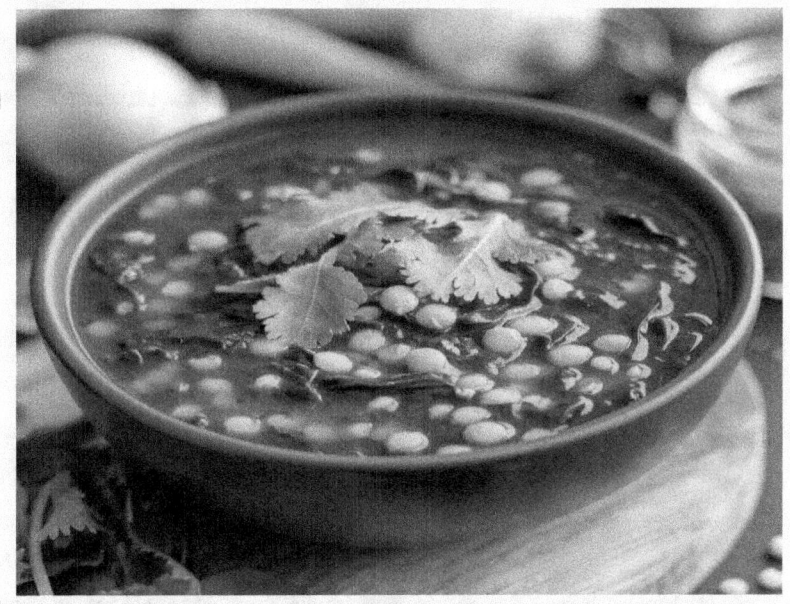

Preparation Method

- Blend spinach, blueberries, strawberries, almond milk, and chia seeds until smooth. Serve immediately.

Nutritional Value

- Calories: 140 kcal

  Protein: 3g

  Carbohydrates: 27g

  Fats: 3g

  Fiber: 8g

  Anti-inflammatory components: Spinach, berries, and chia seeds

Grilled Salmon with Steamed Asparagus

● Ingredients

● 4 oz salmon fillet

1 cup asparagus

1 tablespoon olive oil

Salt and pepper, to taste

Lemon wedge

● Preparation Method

● Grill salmon for 4-5 minutes per side until cooked. Steam asparagus until tender, drizzle with olive oil, and season with salt and pepper. Serve with a lemon wedge.

● Nutritional Value

● Calories: 250 kcal

Protein: 23g

Carbohydrates: 5g

Fats: 16g

Anti-inflammatory components: Omega-3 fatty acids in salmon, olive oil, and asparagus

Turmeric Lentil Soup

Ingredients

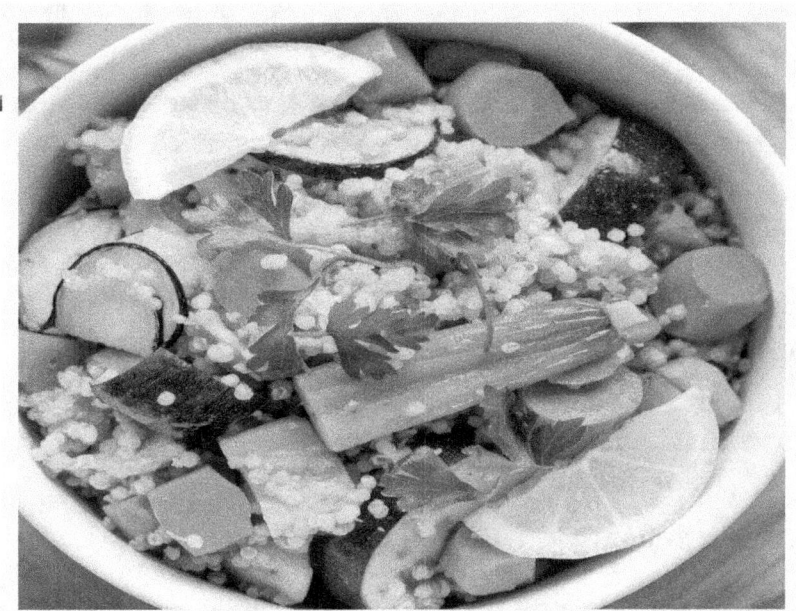

- 1/2 cup red lentils, rinsed

- 2 cups vegetable broth

- 1/2 teaspoon turmeric

- 1 clove garlic, minced

- 1/4 cup diced carrots

- 1/4 cup diced celery

Preparation Method

- In a pot, sauté garlic, carrots, and celery, then add lentils, broth, and turmeric. Simmer for 20 minutes or until lentils are soft.

Nutritional Value

- Calories: 180 kcal

- Protein: 11g

- Carbohydrates: 27g

- Fats: 2g

- Anti-inflammatory components: Turmeric, garlic, and fiber-rich lentils

Kale and Avocado Salad

Ingredients

1 cup chopped kale

1/4 avocado, sliced

1 tablespoon pumpkin seeds

1/2 lemon, juiced

1 tablespoon olive oil

Preparation Method

Massage kale with lemon juice and olive oil until tender. Top with avocado slices and pumpkin seeds.

Nutritional Value

Calories: 170 kcal

Protein: 4g

Carbohydrates: 12g

Fats: 13g

Anti-inflammatory components: Kale, avocado, pumpkin seeds, and olive oil

Ginger Sweet Potato Mash

● Ingredients

● 1 medium sweet potato, peeled and cubed

1/2 teaspoon fresh ginger, grated

1 tablespoon olive oil

● Preparation Method

● Boil sweet potatoes until soft, then mash with grated ginger and olive oil.

● Nutritional Value

● Calories: 150 kcal

Protein: 2g

Carbohydrates: 30g

Fats: 5g

Anti-inflammatory components: Sweet potatoes, ginger, and olive oil

Chickpea and Tomato Stew

● Ingredients

● 1/2 cup chickpeas, cooked

1/4 cup diced tomatoes

1/2 teaspoon cumin

1/2 teaspoon turmeric

1/4 cup chopped spinach

● Preparation Method

● Sauté chickpeas and tomatoes with cumin and turmeric. Add spinach and cook until wilted.

● Nutritional Value

● Calories: 190 kcal

Protein: 8g

Carbohydrates: 26g

Fats: 5g

Anti-inflammatory components: Chickpeas, tomatoes, cumin, and turmeric

Mixed Berry and Chia Seed Pudding

Ingredients

- 1/2 cup unsweetened almond milk

  1 tablespoon chia seeds

  1/4 cup mixed berries

Preparation Method

- Mix chia seeds with almond milk and let sit in the refrigerator for at least 2 hours. Top with

  mixed berries before serving.

Nutritional Value

- Calories: 130 kcal

  Protein: 2g

  Carbohydrates: 14g

  Fats: 5g

  Anti-inflammatory components: Berries and chia seeds

Sautéed Garlic Spinach with Walnuts

● Ingredients

● 1 cup spinach

1 clove garlic, minced

1 tablespoon olive oil

1 tablespoon chopped walnuts

● Preparation Method

● Sauté garlic in olive oil, then add spinach and cook until wilted. Sprinkle with chopped walnuts

before serving.

● Nutritional Value

● Calories: 130 kcal

Protein: 3g

Carbohydrates: 5g

Fats: 11g

Anti-inflammatory components: Spinach, garlic, and walnuts

Avocado and Cucumber Salad with Fresh Herbs

Ingredients

- 1/2 avocado, diced

  1/2 cucumber, sliced

  1 tablespoon fresh parsley, chopped

  1 tablespoon olive oil

  Salt and pepper, to taste

Preparation Method

- Combine avocado, cucumber, and parsley in a bowl. Drizzle with olive oil and season with salt and pepper.

Nutritional Value

- Calories: 180 kcal

  Protein: 2g

  Carbohydrates: 10g

  Fats: 16g

  Anti-inflammatory components: Avocado, cucumber, parsley, and olive oil

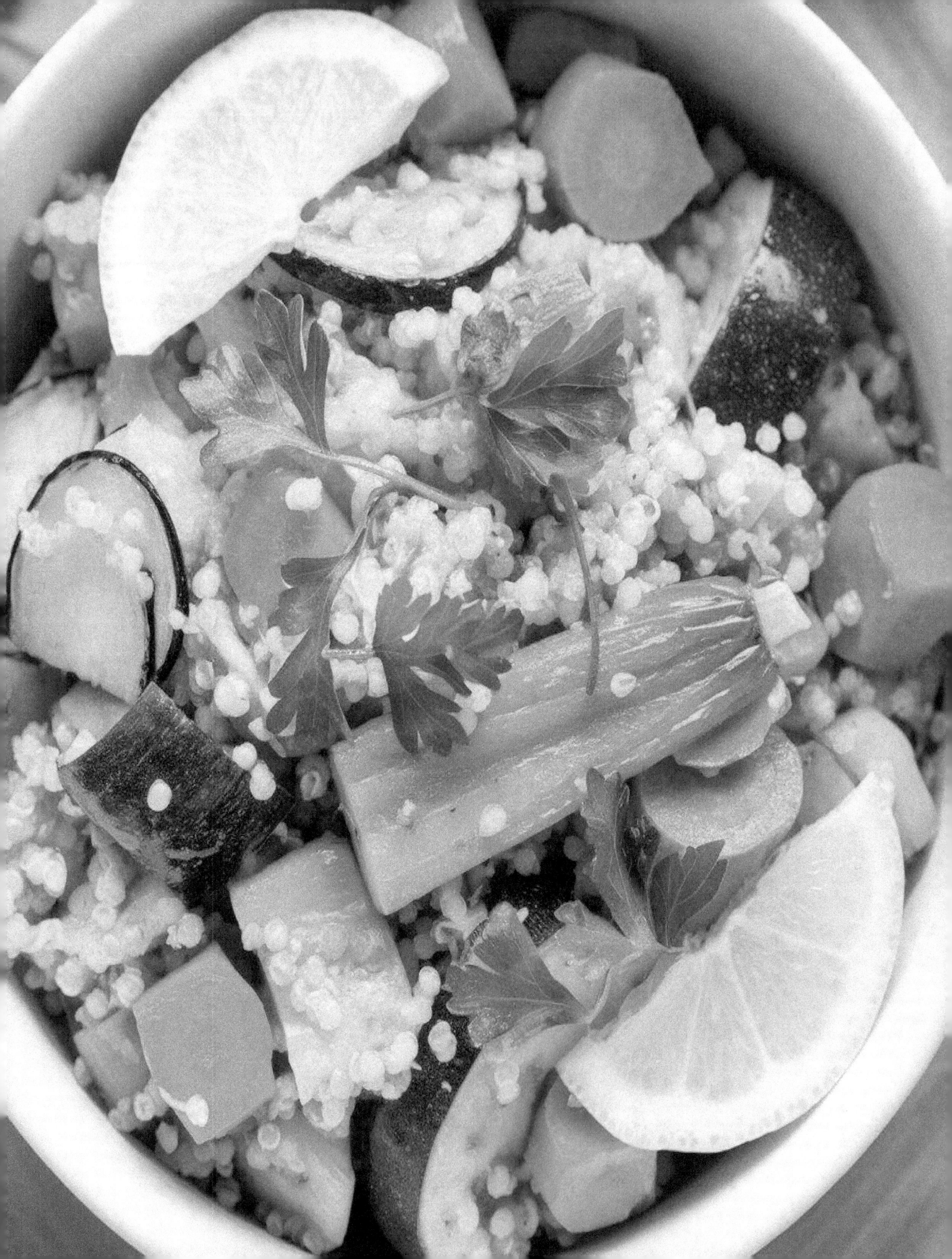

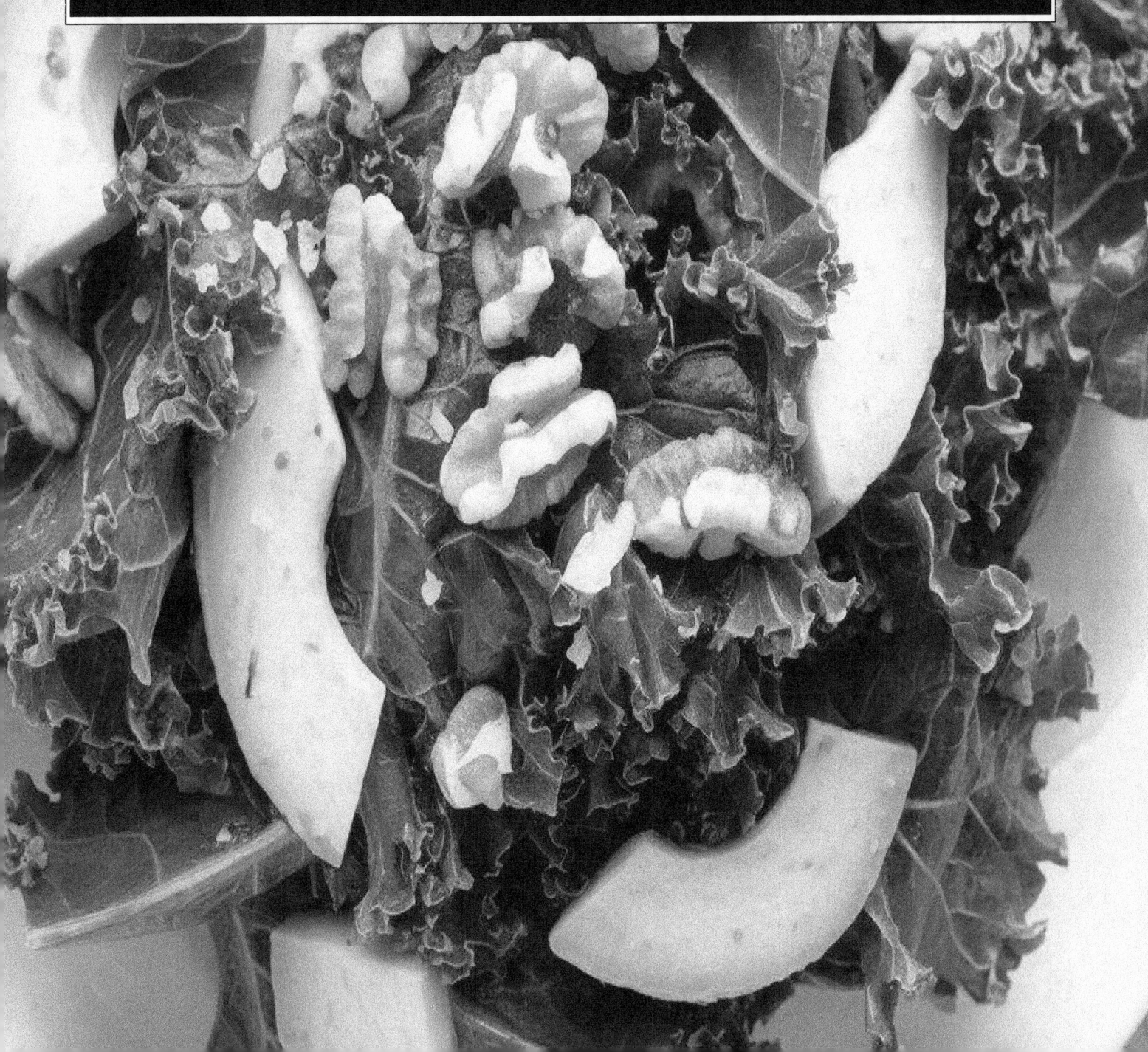

TRACKING YOUR DEVELOPMENT

Monitoring your progress in managing prediabetes is essential to figuring out what works best for you and making the required corrections as you go. Keeping track of your progress keeps you motivated, accountable, and able to appreciate the gains that come with leading a healthy lifestyle. This chapter will cover practical strategies for tracking your physical and mental health, evaluating your eating patterns, and monitoring your blood sugar levels.

The Value of Monitoring Blood Glucose

Monitoring your blood sugar gives you a clear picture of how your body is reacting to changes in your lifestyle. Understanding how diet, exercise, stress, and sleep affect your blood sugar levels is made easier with regular monitoring. You can proactively modify your diet, exercise regimen, and other habits by observing trends in your blood sugar levels.

Blood Glucose Testing Types

The Fasting Blood Sugar (FBS) test determines blood sugar levels following an 8–12 hour fast. It can be performed at home or during regular checkups with the doctor and is useful for determining baseline glucose levels.

PPS, or postprandial blood sugar: This test, which is administered two hours after eating, demonstrates how food affects blood sugar levels. It's a useful tool for tracking the impact of particular meals or snacks.

Glycated hemoglobin, or HbA1c: This test provides a thorough picture of your blood sugar management by calculating your average blood sugar levels over the last three months. Although it is typically completed during doctor's appointments, monitoring it on a regular basis provides important information on long-term development.

Advice for Efficient Blood Sugar Monitoring

Establish a Timetable: Begin with daily tracking and make adjustments according to your lifestyle and results. To evaluate the influence of meals, many people find it useful to test in the morning (fasting) and sometimes after meals.

Maintain a Record: You can identify patterns and triggers by keeping track of your blood glucose levels, whether on paper or using a smartphone app, along with notes about your meals, activity, and emotions.

Evaluating Your Food Practices

Monitoring your food intake involves more than just keeping track of calories or carbohydrates; it also entails knowing how your decisions impact your blood sugar, energy levels, and general health. You can identify areas for improvement and reinforce positive improvements by evaluating your diet.

Techniques for Food Tracking

Keep a daily food journal in which you record all of your meals, their portions, and your feelings both before and after. This might help you identify when you tend to make healthier or less healthy decisions and highlight items that raise blood sugar levels.

Pay Attention to Macronutrient Balance: Take note of the ratios of fats, proteins, and carbohydrates in your meals. Energy levels are maintained and glucose spikes are avoided with balanced macronutrients.

Reflections on Mindful Eating: Keep track of your eating habits, motivations, and emotions. You can address emotional and stress-related eating patterns by identifying them because they can affect blood sugar and progress.

Monitoring Exercise

Exercise is essential for managing weight and blood sugar levels. Frequent exercise increases insulin sensitivity, which facilitates glucose uptake by your cells. You can make sure you're meeting your objectives and maintaining consistency by keeping track of your workouts.

Tips for Tracking Exercise

Establish Weekly Objectives: Strive for a combination of strength training and aerobic exercises (such as swimming, riding, or walking). You can clearly see how committed you are by keeping track of both duration and intensity.

Track Your Development: Keep track of your activities, duration, and post-exercise feelings using a notebook, pedometer, or fitness app. Strength, endurance, and even blood glucose stability will probably improve with time.

Honor Little Victories: Monitoring little gains, such as being able to walk farther or lift more weight, can increase desire and demonstrate the general health advantages of exercise.

Assessing Stress and Sleep

Blood sugar control is impacted by both stress and sleep. Cortisol, a hormone that raises blood sugar levels, can be elevated by stress and inadequate sleep. A crucial component of controlling prediabetes is keeping an eye on these areas.

Advice for Tracking Stress and Sleep

Sleep Journal: Keep track of your bedtime, wake-up time, and any nighttime awakenings. Quality is equally as important as quantity, so try to get 7–9 hours each night and see how you feel in the morning.

Stress Log: Record your everyday stress levels and the things that make them happen. You can find reoccurring stressors and think about strategies to deal with them by setting aside a short period of time each evening to write down your feelings during the day.

Self-Care Practice: Keep an eye on your hobbies, meditation, and deep breathing exercises. Frequent self-care lowers stress and may help blood sugar levels stay more steady.

Examining Your Development and Establishing Objectives

Setting reasonable goals and staying on course are facilitated by routinely assessing your progress. Take some time every few weeks to evaluate your mental well-being, physical activity, food habits, and blood glucose levels.

Establishing and Modifying Objectives

Short-term objectives can be cutting less on sugary snacks, walking for an additional ten minutes each day, or experimenting with new low-glycemic dishes. Setting small, clear objectives fosters the development of enduring habits.

Long-Term Objectives: Consider your desired state after six months or a year. Achieving stable energy levels, sticking to a regular exercise schedule, or hitting a target HbA1c level are a few examples of these objectives.

Adapt as necessary: Don't be scared to review and modify your objectives. Managing prediabetes is a journey, and the secret to figuring out what works best for you is flexibility.

One powerful strategy to manage your prediabetes is to keep track of your progress. You can better understand how these factors affect your health by monitoring your blood glucose levels, food, exercise, sleep, and stress levels. Keep in mind that every little step forward counts and advances you toward your objectives.

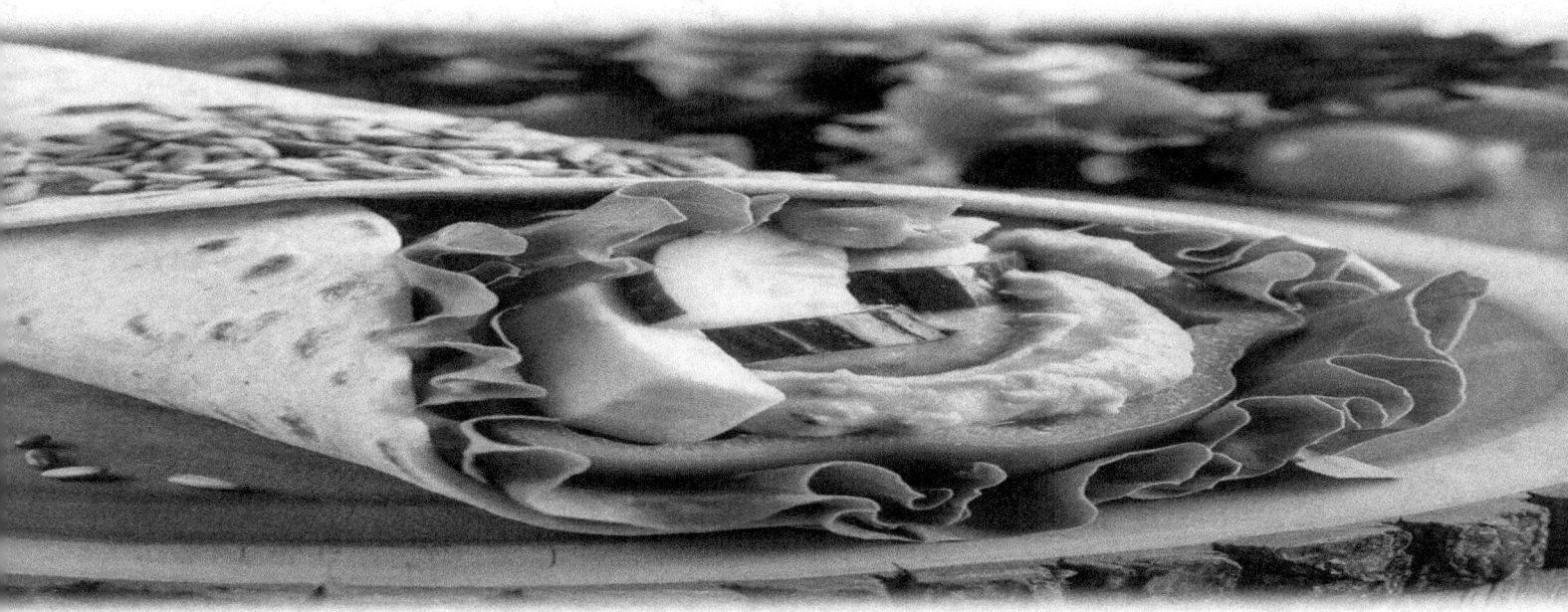

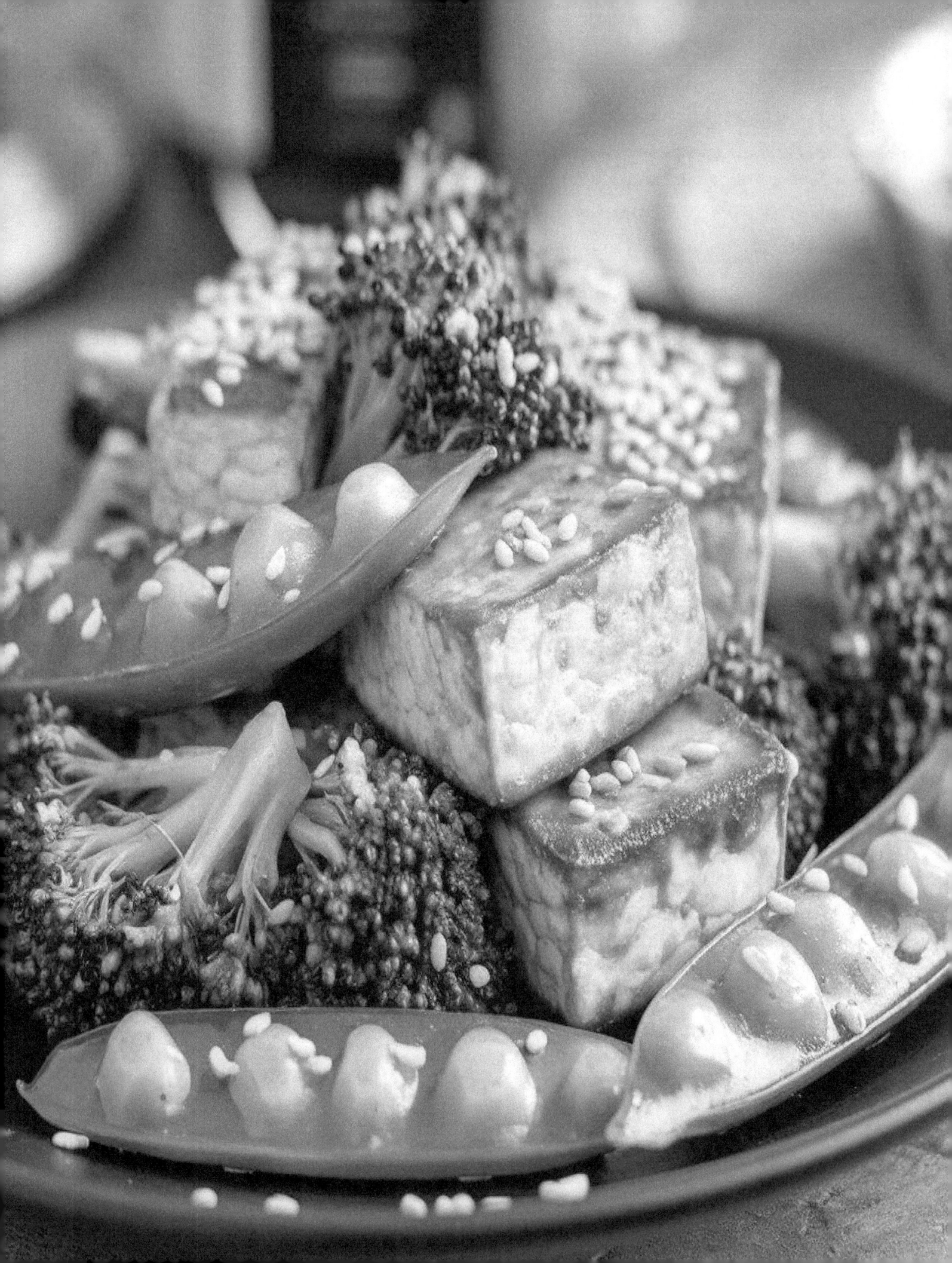

THE EXCEPTIONALLY

SIMPLE

PREDIABETES

ACTION PLAN

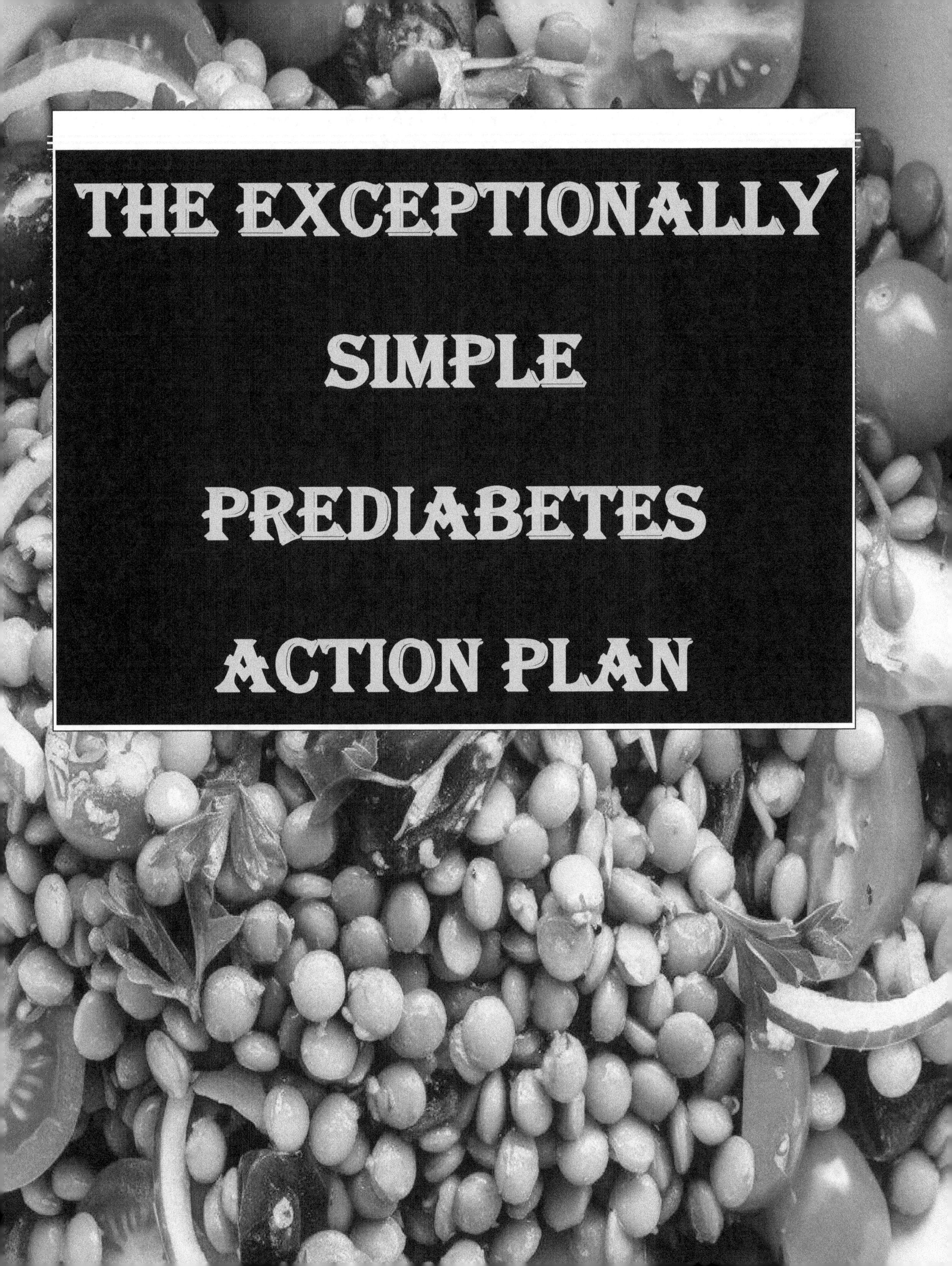

Starting a prediabetes management path is a strong commitment to your health and wellbeing. Even while breaking bad habits can seem overwhelming, a well-defined plan can make the process easier and help you make your goals a reality. This chapter will walk you through developing a customized plan, establishing reasonable objectives, and turning your health-related behavior into a lifetime commitment.

Making a Customized Strategy

A strategy that fits your own requirements, tastes, and way of life is essential for long-term success. There is rarely a one-size-fits-all strategy for managing prediabetes. The factors that have the greatest effects on blood sugar and general health—diet, exercise, stress reduction, and sleep—should be the main focus of your customized plan.

Analyze Your Present Habits: Start by evaluating your way of life. For a week, keep a notebook to record your stress levels, sleep, physical activity, and dietary habits. Knowing where you are at this moment can assist you identify the areas that require the greatest attention.

Dietary Changes: Whole foods, fiber, and balanced macronutrients are key components of a prediabetes-friendly diet. Make tiny, doable adjustments at first, such as increasing the amount of veggies in your diet, opting for whole grains rather than refined ones, and incorporating lean proteins into each meal. To avoid spikes, use low-glycemic options if you enjoy carbohydrates.

Exercise Routine: Getting regular exercise improves insulin sensitivity and aids in blood sugar regulation. Consistency is crucial, so pick something you enjoy doing. Try to get in at least 150 minutes a week of moderate-intensity exercise, which should include both strength training and cardio (such as walking or biking).

Stress and Sleep Management: Excessive stress and restless nights can raise cortisol levels, which can affect blood sugar levels. Include stress-relieving pursuits like yoga, meditation, or a favorite pastime, and establish a consistent sleep routine with a goal of 7 to 9 hours each night.

Frequent Monitoring: Keep tabs on your blood pressure, weight, cholesterol, and blood sugar levels, among other health indicators. Monitoring provides you with important information about your development and enables you to observe how your body reacts to changes.

Establishing Achievable, Realistic Goals

Setting attainable goals is essential for any lifestyle adjustment. Setting and achieving goals gives you focus, direction, and a sense of success. Here's a method for creating objectives that encourage long-term improvements in health:

Establish Specific, Measurable Goals: Clearly state your objectives and provide quantifiable standards for success. Set a goal like "I'll include a serving of vegetables in each meal this week" rather than just "I want to eat healthier."

Divide Long-Term Objectives into Short-Term phases: Although big objectives may appear overwhelming, they are easier to handle when divided into weekly or monthly phases. If your long-term objective is to work out five days a week, for instance, start with three days and work your way up.

Concentrate on Making Small, Sustainable Changes: Long-term success depends on consistency. Aiming for a radical change in lifestyle all at once may result in burnout. Start with manageable, incremental changes, such as increasing your daily exercise time by ten minutes or replacing a sugary snack with a piece of fruit.

Honor Milestones: Acknowledge and commemorate your advancements along the path. Positive reinforcement increases motivation and strengthens good habits. Examples of this include rewarding yourself with something you enjoy or sharing your accomplishments with a friend or family member.

Developing a Lifelong Interest in Health

Adopting a lifestyle that promotes long-term health is crucial to controlling prediabetes. Consider this a permanent commitment that enhances your general well-being rather than concentrating on limitations or temporary objectives.

Develop a Positive Attitude: The success of any health journey is greatly influenced by your attitude. Consider lifestyle modifications as chances to feel better, have more energy, and lower your risk of developing health issues in the future rather than as limitations. Accept the advantages that come with each new habit.

Create a Support System: Support and accountability can be obtained via a network of friends, family, or even an online community. Talk to those who can help you achieve your goals, and think about joining forces with a friend who shares your objectives.

Regularly Reevaluate: As you make progress, reflect on your progress and adapt as necessary. Your demands and tastes will change as your life circumstances do. To stay in line with your personal and health objectives, review your goals from time to time and don't be scared to make changes to your plan.

Continue Your Education: Learning about health is a lifelong journey. Keep up with the latest findings, nutritious recipes, and fitness methods that may help you. Being informed will empower you and keep you inspired and involved in your health journey.

Allow for Flexibility: Perfection isn't the aim, and life will always have its ups and downs. Be flexible without feeling guilty. The important thing is to get back to your healthy routines without giving up.

You will be able to control prediabetes and enhance your health with a customized, practical approach that is based on attainable objectives and a lifetime commitment. You may develop a sustainable lifestyle that improves your well-being and promotes long-term health by incorporating these adjustments gradually. Keep in mind that each constructive adjustment you make is a step closer to a healthy future.

CONCLUSION

Managing prediabetes is not just about numbers or a checklist of changes; it's about crafting a sustainable, fulfilling lifestyle that supports your health and well-being. Throughout this book, we've explored the essentials of prediabetes management, from understanding blood glucose and adopting healthier food choices to integrating exercise, managing stress, and setting realistic goals. Each chapter has been a guide to creating a balanced, personalized approach that empowers you to take control of your health with confidence.

As you move forward, remember that the journey to a healthier you is a gradual process. Small steps, taken consistently, yield the greatest impact. Monitoring your progress and making adjustments based on your body's responses will help you stay on track. This journey isn't about perfection but about finding the balance that works best for you.

Take pride in each positive choice, each small milestone, and every commitment you make to a healthier lifestyle. Equip yourself with knowledge, surround yourself with support, and embrace the flexibility to grow and adapt as your needs evolve. With patience and persistence, you'll build habits that not only help manage prediabetes but also enrich your life with energy, strength, and resilience. Here's to a lifelong commitment to health and wellness—one step at a time.

SHOPPING/GROCERY LIST

Food Category	Recommended Foods	Tips for Selection
Whole Grains	Quinoa, brown rice, oats, whole wheat bread	Choose whole grain options with minimal processing. Look for "100% whole grain" labels.
Fruits	Berries (blueberries, strawberries), apples, pears, oranges	Opt for fresh or frozen fruits without added sugars. Choose whole fruits over juices.
Vegetables	Leafy greens (spinach, kale), broccoli, carrots, bell peppers	Select a variety of colors for a range of nutrients. Buy fresh, frozen, or canned (low sodium) options.
Legumes	Lentils, chickpeas, black beans, kidney beans	Choose canned versions with no added sugars or salt. Dried legumes are also a great option.
Lean Proteins	Chicken breast, turkey, fish (salmon, tuna), tofu, tempeh	Look for skinless poultry and wild-caught fish. Choose low-fat dairy or plant-based options.
Healthy Fats	Avocados, olive oil, nuts (almonds, walnuts), seeds (chia, flax)	Select unsalted nuts and seeds. Use extra virgin olive oil for cooking and dressings.
Dairy Alternatives	Unsweetened almond milk, coconut yogurt, low-fat cheese	Look for options without added sugars. Choose fortified alternatives for added nutrients.
Herbs and Spices	Basil, oregano, turmeric, cinnamon	Fresh or dried options can enhance flavor without added sugars or sodium. Opt for organic when possible.
Snacks	Hummus, Greek yogurt, air-popped popcorn, dark chocolate (70% cocoa or higher)	Choose snacks low in added sugars and unhealthy fats. Read labels for portion sizes.
Beverages	Water, herbal tea, unsweetened iced tea	Limit sugary drinks and fruit juices. Infuse water with fruits for flavor without added sugars.

40 DAYS ACTIVE

MEAL PLAN

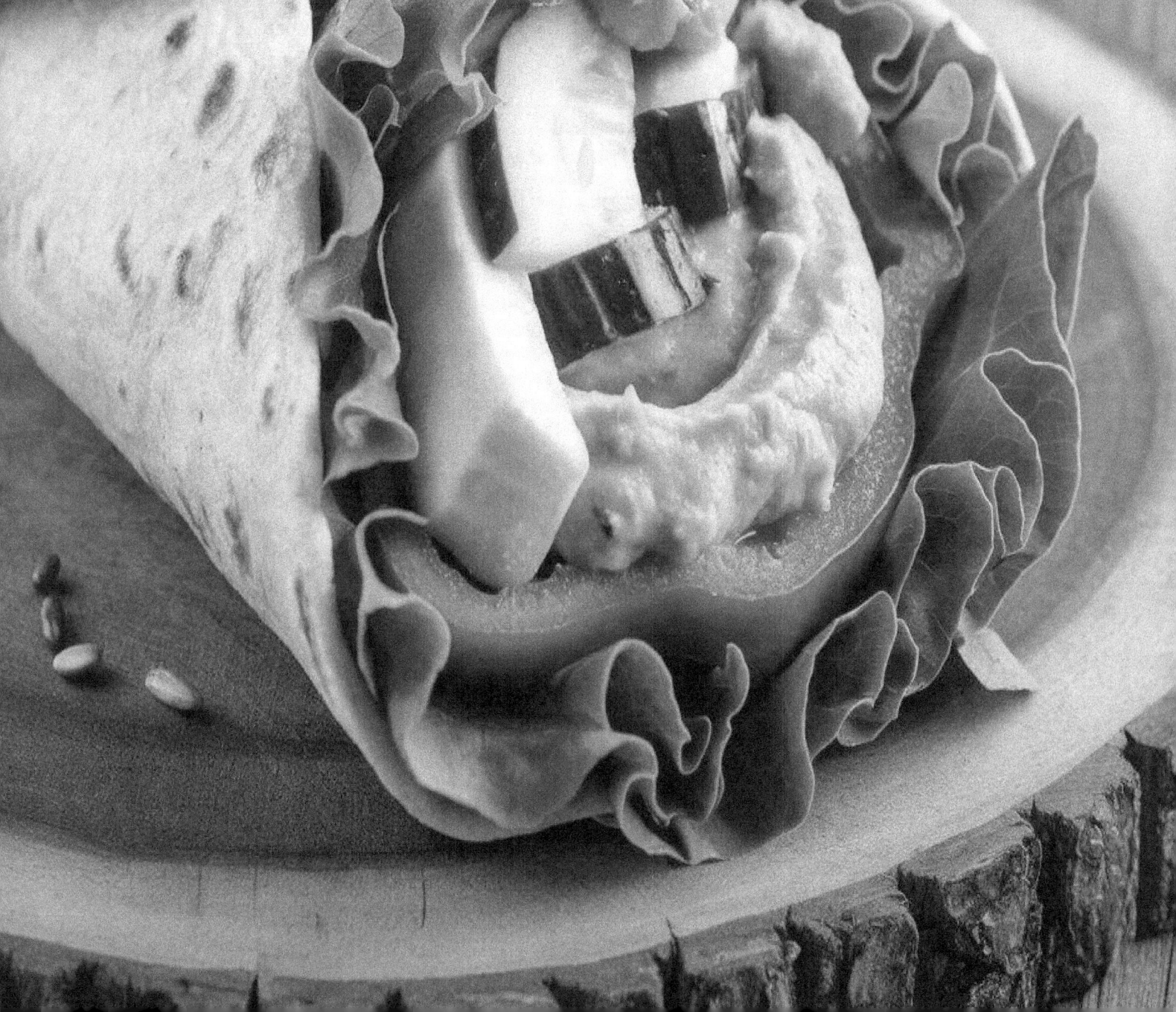

Day	Breakfast	Lunch	Dinner	Snacks
1	Oatmeal with berries	Quinoa salad with chickpeas	Grilled chicken with steamed broccoli	Greek yogurt with nuts
2	Scrambled eggs with spinach	Turkey wrap in whole grain tortilla	Baked salmon with asparagus	Apple slices with almond butter
3	Greek yogurt with flaxseed	Lentil soup	Stir-fried tofu with mixed vegetables	Carrot sticks with hummus
4	Smoothie with spinach and banana	Brown rice with black beans	Grilled shrimp with quinoa	Celery with peanut butter
5	Whole grain toast with avocado	Spinach salad with grilled chicken	Stuffed bell peppers with quinoa	Cottage cheese with pineapple
6	Chia seed pudding with berries	Mediterranean quinoa salad	Zucchini noodles with marinara sauce	Mixed nuts
7	Omelet with tomatoes and onions	Hummus with whole grain pita	Baked tilapia with roasted vegetables	Dark chocolate (small piece)
8	Smoothie with almond milk and berries	Turkey and veggie stir-fry	Grilled vegetable kebabs	Greek yogurt with berries
9	Overnight oats with chia seeds	Quinoa and black bean salad	Baked chicken with sweet potatoes	Apple with cheese
10	Whole grain pancakes with fruit	Vegetable soup	Beef stir-fry with broccoli	Cucumber slices with tzatziki
11	Egg and vegetable frittata	Lentil and spinach salad	Grilled pork tenderloin with Brussels sprouts	Sliced bell peppers with guacamole
12	Yogurt with nuts and seeds	Chickpea salad with cucumber	Roasted chicken with cauliflower	Berries with cottage cheese
13	Smoothie with spinach and protein powder	Brown rice with grilled vegetables	Quinoa bowl with black beans	Almonds and dried fruit
14	Oatmeal with sliced banana	Tuna salad on mixed greens	Baked salmon with green beans	Hummus with carrot sticks
15	Avocado toast on whole grain bread	Turkey and cheese roll-ups	Veggie stir-fry with tofu	Popcorn (air-popped)
16	Greek yogurt with honey and berries	Whole grain wrap with veggies	Chicken fajitas with bell peppers	Trail mix (unsweetened)
17	Chia seed pudding with almond milk	Spinach and feta salad	Shrimp tacos in lettuce wraps	Dark chocolate (small piece)
18	Smoothie with kale and mango	Quinoa bowl with roasted veggies	Beef and vegetable kabobs	Apple slices with almond butter
19	Scrambled eggs with tomatoes	Lentil and quinoa salad	Grilled chicken with asparagus	Greek yogurt with nuts
20	Overnight oats with walnuts	Chickpea and spinach salad	Baked fish with zucchini	Celery with peanut butter
21	Whole grain toast with nut butter	Turkey and vegetable soup	Stir-fried tofu with broccoli	Cucumber slices with tzatziki
22	Omelet with mushrooms and spinach	Quinoa and bean salad	Grilled pork with green beans	Mixed nuts

23	Smoothie with berries and spinach	Mediterranean chickpea salad	Baked chicken with mixed vegetables	Berries with cottage cheese
24	Yogurt with chia seeds and fruit	Lentil soup with spinach	Grilled shrimp with quinoa	Hummus with whole grain crackers
25	Oatmeal with apples and cinnamon	Spinach and avocado salad	Veggie stir-fry with tofu	Sliced bell peppers with guacamole
26	Scrambled eggs with avocado	Brown rice and veggie bowl	Stuffed bell peppers with quinoa	Dark chocolate (small piece)
27	Whole grain pancakes with fruit	Turkey and vegetable wrap	Grilled chicken with sweet potatoes	Almonds and dried fruit
28	Smoothie with spinach and protein powder	Chickpea salad with cucumber	Baked fish with roasted vegetables	Greek yogurt with berries
29	Chia seed pudding with berries	Lentil and spinach salad	Grilled pork with Brussels sprouts	Popcorn (air-popped)
30	Oatmeal with sliced banana	Tuna salad on mixed greens	Beef stir-fry with broccoli	Sliced bell peppers with tzatziki
31	Avocado toast on whole grain bread	Quinoa bowl with black beans	Veggie stir-fry with tofu	Carrot sticks with hummus
32	Greek yogurt with honey and walnuts	Vegetable soup	Chicken fajitas with bell peppers	Dark chocolate (small piece)
33	Smoothie with kale and mango	Brown rice with grilled vegetables	Baked chicken with asparagus	Hummus with carrot sticks
34	Omelet with mushrooms and spinach	Lentil soup with spinach	Grilled shrimp with quinoa	Greek yogurt with nuts
35	Overnight oats with walnuts	Spinach and feta salad	Baked fish with zucchini	Apple with cheese
36	Whole grain toast with nut butter	Turkey and vegetable soup	Stuffed bell peppers with quinoa	Cucumber slices with tzatziki
37	Smoothie with spinach and protein powder	Chickpea salad with cucumber	Grilled chicken with sweet potatoes	Almonds and dried fruit
38	Chia seed pudding with berries	Lentil and quinoa salad	Grilled pork with green beans	Berries with cottage cheese
39	Oatmeal with apples and cinnamon	Tuna salad on mixed greens	Veggie stir-fry with tofu	Sliced bell peppers with guacamole
40	Avocado toast on whole grain bread	Quinoa bowl with black beans	Grilled chicken with asparagus	Popcorn (air-popped)